SAILING THROUGH
THE STORMS OF
SEIZURES

SAILING THROUGH
THE STORMS OF
SEIZURES

Living with Epilepsy, Recovering from
Brain Surgery, and Being a Caregiver

JON SADLER

Print information available on the last page.

Rev. date: 06/23/2018

To order additional copies of this book, contact:
Xlibris
1-888-795-4274
www.Xlibris.com
Orders@Xlibris.com
773194

Hope we have as an anchor of the soul.

—Hebrews 6:19 New King James Version and the State Seal of Rhode Island

The tiniest sense of hope is the anchor that can overcome negative thoughts.

"For all those dealing with seizure disorders."

Contents

Introduction

My father told me I should never tell anyone I have epilepsy. He knew there would be times when people would label me, and I would be discriminated against simply because my brain would shut down on occasion. It was 1979, my sophomore year in college, and I was studying to be a civil engineer. He was right in many ways; I would learn firsthand about the stigmas associated with having seizures. To pull me through, I made a contract with God: I asked for twenty years of control over my seizures. God never signed the contract; nevertheless, hope had been instilled in me.

My seizures were controlled for many years through medication. When I had a breakthrough seizure, there seemed to be a new medication available, and the seizures were under control for a few more years. I was able to work as an engineer and eventually became a project manager. My level of responsibility and the projects I was involved with were unique and important.

I was married and had two children. Every time I accomplished something important, through work or family, there was the setback of a seizure. Eventually, my seizures dominated my life; they reached the stage of being intractable and being untreatable. I went from a seizure every few years to several per week. Surgery involving the removal of a section of my brain—the control center of my engineering skills—was the only option left.

I kept asking God why. The answer rarely came immediately. For me this required thirty-five years—the time it would take to have enough experience to help other people with epilepsy. The answer came through a phone call from a colleague whose child had intractable seizures; he had no hope. Everything I had experienced with my epilepsy now had meaning.

This was my *ah-ha* moment—a new beginning for me. Hope had been instilled in me; now it was time to instill hope in others. I became a mentor in the Epilepsy Foundation, helping people diagnosed with epilepsy and their families. Then my counselor challenged me to go back to school to obtain a Master's Degree in Pastoral Counseling. This seemed impossible, for my memory was damaged and recall very poor.

Through my studies, I learned more about the brain and found many other situations people faced similar to myself—being broken, hopeless, and filled with anxiety and despair. Through my internship as a counselor, I worked with people dealing with addictions and others with brain injury. My experience enabled me to quickly associate with them and work with them. I did not share my story; I simply could associate in an effective manner.

Being a caregiver for a person you love and who suffers from a seizure disorder is troubling and strenuous, both physically and mentally. I became the caregiver when the person I love started having complex seizures. I have seen many people have seizures; it is much different when the person you love is having one. Driven by my emotions, I started to overreact and needed to talk to another person who was a caregiver.

I often struggled with being open to others about myself. Now, in spite of what my father had told me, it is time to share my experience—to help those who are struggling with or know someone who is dealing with epilepsy, brain injury, addiction, or some other disease or accident. The foundation I share for survival and recovery is based on the three fundamentals identified by a disciple over two thousand years ago: perseverance, faith, and hope.

Acknowledgements

This book is about how I have lived with epilepsy for over fifty years. The people and events in this book are real. There were many people who I have had contact with who helped me live with my fears or provided medical treatment. I cannot remember all the names, and maybe that is a good thing for I want to make sure their privacy is maintained. For those I do remember, I have changed many of the names; the exception is with family and those whose full names are presented.

The people referenced in my clinical work may consist of a summary of a group of people I worked or associated with. In these cases, they are referenced with pronouns.

The institutions and agencies mentioned truly exist, and the contact information is provided at the end to the book. Further information concerning education, treatment, and chat groups are available through these agencies.

There were several people who helped me with this book. Many were classmates who told me to, "Share my story". Others were people suffering with seizures; one of whom was Marla, who has maintained a positive outlook, and shared her God given talents as a mentor, editor, and friend. Another was Lori, who taught me what it is like to be the caregiver of someone you love.

Section 1

Understanding Epilepsy

Chapter 1

The Brain and Seizures

Epilepsy is not a punishment on a person or their family for something they have done. It is a condition of the brain requiring respect, knowledge, and care. Control comes through the ability to live without the fear of rejection.

Our brain is the most fascinating component of our bodies. It is the center of our nervous system, consisting of over a trillion neurons, and sends electrical impulses throughout our body. It activates and monitors our heart, lungs, digestive system, and the dilation of our eyes. The sounds we hear are transferred into electrical impulses in our ears and transferred to a section of our brain for processing. It is the center of how we feel about ourselves, controlling our emotions. It is the master control center.

We hear many sounds around us and control what we want to remember. Various sounds become background noise, as the mind defines what we want to hear. Similarly, smell and taste is processed through another part of the brain. The brain responds accordingly to what it likes and doesn't like. The nervous system is an intricate wiring system running throughout the body. Everything we touch and feel is transmitted through the nerves and processed in the brain. Pain is vital to knowing there is something wrong or something is physically hurting a part of the body. Feeling pain and the intensity is controlled in the brain.

Vision is based on the light contacting our eyes and contacting through the nervous system that is controlled from the back of the brain. The memory part of the brain identifies the objects and colors we see.

What is even more interesting is how the information is processed and how the necessity to remember on short-term or long-term basis is determined; for instance, remembering the quote in a movie yet not recalling the title. How can we do so well on a quiz yet not recall the information on the final exam? Why do many of us struggle with remembering names?

Then there are the emotions—those feelings and responses to what happens around us. For some of us, crying or laughing comes at an appropriate time, and we fit in with the rest of the group. Not everyone responds the same way. A few cry when others laugh, and for some, they do not know what it is like to do either.

The center of the brain that controls fear is known as the amygdala. It is the size of a large pea, and there are two of them—one in the left and one in the right hemisphere of the brain. How does one learn to control feelings, especially when they are overwhelmed by them? When fear becomes the dominating feeling, it takes one into the dark side of life, feeding depression and anxiety and preventing a person from moving forward.

Epilepsy

As a mentor and counselor, I am often asked, "What is epilepsy?" and "What is the cause?" Epilepsy is diagnosed when a person has two or more seizures that are not considered a side effect to a medication. A seizure is an electrical storm in a part of the brain that causes sections to stop working temporarily. It may affect a small part of the brain or all of it. During a seizure, various sections of the brain are impacted, and functional abilities are lost or distorted. It affects many people as their abilities are limited by their ignorance and fear of a seizure, whether they are the person with epilepsy, their caregiver, or the people with whom they come in contact.

Epilepsy is a seizure disorder that has been known for thousands of years. Sophocles wrote of it, and people such as Alexander the Great and Julius Caesar had epilepsy. In ancient Roman society, a person with epilepsy was highly respected because seizures were thought to be a way the gods communicated with people. Caesar's greatest fear when leading men into battle was not the outcome of the battle; it was having a seizure that would make him incapable of leading his men.

In the Middle Ages, and in some cultures today, people were isolated from others for fear of seizures spreading. Epileptics were considered possessed by demons, and exorcism was practiced to make the demons leave the body. In reality, there is no demon, no possession, and no punishment by a god.

Medical Perspective

From a medical perspective, epilepsy is when there is more than one seizure with a neurological disorder in the brain. The cause is often unknown; however, in many cases, the cause may be from a high fever, infection, or head injury. These situations often cause enough injury to leave lesions (similar to scars) within the brain. A medial temporal lobe seizure is one of the most common forms of epilepsy. It is most often caused by a major injury such as meningitis or head trauma.

As a young child or adolescent, it is not unusual for the brain to outgrow or develop in the problem area where the neurons are overloaded or the chemistry becomes balanced, resulting in no more seizures. This often takes years, and the person may never have another seizure. However, prolonged seizures occurring prior to the age of four and followed with additional head injury creates more scarring in the brain, resulting in seizures forming by the teenage years.

With older adults, the brain aging and degenerating may be the onset. A lack of blood flow to the brain caused by a heart defect or the arteries from the heart becoming restricted may cause a seizure, especially in women.

Seizure Triggers

Changes in medication levels are a common cause for breakthrough seizures; therefore, a person must take it daily as directed by their physicians without missing dosages to maintain the appropriate blood. Missing doses increases the risk of having a seizure, especially when a person does not believe they need it anymore. It is also important to get medication levels checked several times a year for a person's metabolism changes as they age. Being on the same medication for many years may lead to a decrease in the amount required to keep the same blood level.

The side effects of medications can be minimal to some, or it can be incapacitating or physically harming to others. Prior to starting a medication, the doctor should discuss the side effects with the patient. If the medication affects the personality, which is not unusual, the doctor should be notified immediately, and options should be discussed. There have been cases where a spouse or parent could no longer relate to their loved one due to the negative changes in personality. The happy and energetic person they knew was now angry or severely depressed since being on a medication.

Changes in stress and anxiety levels are a leading cause of seizures. There are two basic forms or stress on the body—the physical and mental. High levels of physical stress often cause seizures as the body becomes dehydrated and chemically imbalanced, especially when such stress is not occurring on a regular basis, such as overexertion when starting an exercise program. Exercise programs are very healthy for most people and effective in lowering physical and mental stress levels. However, starting slow and building up is necessary for anyone, even if they do not have to be concerned with having a seizure.

Increases and decreases in mental stress cause a change within the brain that affects the entire body. It is known that an increase in stress is a tripping point for a seizure, especially as a person begins to dramatize the situation, enabling their fears to increase. This is often exacerbated by the outcomes they imagine. When such stressors are resolved, the fears go away, and the brain slows down as the dramatization ends. These shifts decrease the impulses in the brain. And for some people, they are the triggers to their seizures.

Sleep deprivation is another common trigger. If a person cannot sleep, they should rest regardless. Staying away from caffeine and sugar is helpful. Worrying about the amount of sleep one gets often will keep a person awake. Simply rest the body and the brain. If the brain is busy with thoughts, write them down so one does not have to remember them anymore, and they can be addressed the next day. Let nature take its course.

Stress and sleep deprivation lead to exhaustion—another key trigger to seizures. Exhaustion is when the body has no energy and is exacerbated with the inability to think clearly. Our bodies and minds need rest and need to recharge naturally.

Eating regularly and consuming fluids affects the body's chemistry and plays a role in seizure activity. Dehydration is a key factor, and eating three meals a day is important, especially meals that consist of foods that are nutritious. Fast-food hamburgers were a problem for me, so I make sure I get good quality foods with little to no preservatives. Drinking fluids is essential; water and drinks with lower sodium is very helpful.

For some women with epilepsy, their initial seizure occurred when they started having menstrual cycles. Although they may have a seizure at any time, they tend to be most susceptible just prior to menses.[1] Menopause has been a time when some women start having seizures as their body chemistry changes.

A seizure triggered by flashing light is known as photosensitive epilepsy. It is usually associated with a genetic form of epilepsy and is a rare condition. Many children love to play video games where there is a sequence of lights flashing in the two-dimensional view of the TV screen, enhanced to appear to be three-dimensional.

---

[1]	Seizures associated with the menstrual period are usually due to drops in progesterone, which reduces seizures in the luteal phase right before menses. Progesterone replacement didn't help most women with this trigger.

The brain gets confused, and the flashing lights overwhelm a part that leads to a seizure. The special effects in movies often create similar conditions and may cause a seizure. I quickly learned when to close my eyes as my aura started. Through people I have met, I learned how swimming pools with reflective sunlight caused by the movement of the water are also key seizure triggers. The difficulty in determining photosensitive seizures is how excitement is a trigger, often exacerbated by the nature of video games.

Seizures often start or are triggered by an environmental condition, event, or setting. They may be simple—as the alternating sun/shade associated with travel, such as riding down the highway and the sun shining between trees—or complex, which involves multiple conditions. Traveling to a location away from home creates changes in the environment, including the water consumed, the types and sources of food, air temperature, and time zone. Any one or a combination of these trigger a seizure. The person may be stressed about the reason for the trip and fear the manner of transportation, be it flying or riding in a car. Blood levels of medication may change due to the chemistry of the foods, adapting to time zones, and changes in physical activity. He or she may drink bottled water to help decrease the changes in the chemistry of the water, and reviewing the impact to medication levels with a doctor is very helpful.

Not all triggers may be identified. As the history of an individual's seizures is kept and reviewed, the triggers may be identified and avoided. A person should keep a record of each seizure that includes medications, diet, sleep, and stress during the previous twenty-four hours. There may be a series of events that occur regularly that may be avoided or minimized to reduce the risk.

A Seizure That Is Not Epilepsy

In some cases, a seizure can be a reaction to a new medication, a change in dosage, or a chemical to which a person is exposed. These consist of medications associated with treating another part of the body and not for seizures.

I oversaw a seminar for thirty people on estimating cost and time for construction projects. The woman sitting next to me was asking a question to the instructor when suddenly, she quit talking as her body went completely rigid. Her muscles were so tense that every part of her body was shaking. Her head pounded against the back of the chair, and she lost control of her bladder as she unknowingly urinated onto the floor. I quickly got behind her and placed my hands between her head and the back of the chair to create a buffer so she would not hurt her head. My associate got up and ran toward the door, shouting that he was going to the nurses' office to get help.

The next two minutes were very traumatic for everyone as the seizure continued and the person did not breathe. Her body turned a shade of blue, with her lips becoming deep blue. There was nothing anyone could do during that period. The only part of the chair she had contact with was the front edge with her hips and the top of the back support where her head pounded against my hands. The back edge of her shoes was in contact with the floor as her body was perfectly straight due to all her muscles contracting. Her muscles were so tense they shook, causing her body to jerk in a steady rhythm. Eventually, her body began to go limp, and I could feel her heart beating rapidly through her neck. Yet she still did not breathe. I kept her airway clear by tilting her head back. And just as I was about to breathe into her mouth, she coughed and took a deep breath. I can still replay it in my mind.

Her eyes began to wander as she tried to figure out where she was and what had happened. Another associate helped me pull her back onto the chair. About this time, the nurse arrived with a wheelchair and took care of the woman. We later learned she never had a seizure before, and the cause was due to a change in a medication. She was never diagnosed with epilepsy.

After the nurse left, I looked at the instructor who had been talking to the woman when she had the seizure. My immediate response was "We can get started again." It was then I realized he was pale and had not moved since the seizure began. He was staring at her empty chair. At this point, I told everyone, "Let's take a break and talk about what had happened." First aid, through education, was required for the instructor and several people attending the seminar.

I walked up to the instructor and quietly asked him if he was OK. He kept staring at the chair. I kept a calm voice and told him what he witnessed was the woman having a seizure. As I discussed what he saw, he looked at me and turned his body to face me. He calmed down as I told him the woman was going to be fine and was with the nursing staff. When people saw and heard what I was doing, they approached the stage, wanting to learn more to settle their fears with what they witnessed. Everyone was surprised when they learned I have epilepsy and recover from seizures, and they were reassured when I suggested we continue the class.

After class, one of the men told me he has a twenty-year-old son with epilepsy. Like myself, the child had a high fever at the age of five. His fever lasted considerably longer than mine and caused more damage to the same section of his brain. In many ways, he remained a five-year-old for his mental development was severely damaged. We kept in touch for over fifteen years.

The Brain

The brain is a network of wires known as neurons and is the control center of the entire body. It consistently develops and changes to meet the requirements of what it is programmed to do. In early childhood, it develops the fundamentals in life such as eating, tasting, talking, identifying, to name a few. It is the actual connection or sequencing of neurons as they come together or detach to create the memory of an event or emotion. It is fascinating to watch infants wanting to touch and taste everything. When they do not like how hot or cold the item is or how it tastes, they remember not to touch or taste them again. Although someone can tell them what will happen, it will not register in the brain until they witness it. This often continues well into early adulthood. This follows the old cliché of "Most people don't believe the paint is wet until you touch it."

In the adolescent stage, there are more changes as the child learns to associate with people outside the home and discover their interests and abilities. Often the answers to a question, especially when asked by a parent, is a delayed "Yes," "No," or "I don't know." They delay responding as they search through their brains for the answers. The problem is, many children cannot find it because their brains are going through a significant change in development.

Brain Components

The brain has five major components referred to as lobes. Each lobe performs a basic function with body senses and memory. The frontal lobe is the basis of memory, behavior, movement, and intelligence. The parietal lobe is the center of language, sensation, and reading. At the back of the brain is the optical lobe, and it is associated with vision. The cerebellum is at the base of the brain and controls balance and coordination. The center of behavior, hearing, speech, vision, and memory is the focus of the temporal lobe.

There is a series of structures and glands that tie the lobes together and affect various components of the body. The limbic system is the center of emotions and includes the amygdala, hippocampus, hypothalamus, and thalamus. The amygdala controls rage and emotional responses, and the hippocampus affects memory. We have right and left hippocampi and amygdala and can usually remove one without changes in effect; memory for verbal information goes down slightly with removal of the left dominant hippocampus. Like the computer RAM, the hippocampus assorts the information presented through the senses and stores it in the cerebellum. Then, when the need arises, it pulls back the information.

Electrical Storms of a Seizure

The brain is made up of nerve cells which form the outer part of the brain called the cortex. These nerve cells, known as neurons, have transmission fibers called axons that form the deep part of the brain, also called white matter, since they are lined with fat-rich insulation called myelin. Any injury that causes nerve tangles in the cortex can cause abnormal electrical transmission between nerves. When these get synchronized—discharge in rhythm—then seizures consisting of abnormal electrical conduction across the brain's nerves can form.[2]

When a neuron gets overloaded, it passes the impulse onto other neurons. As more neurons become excited, the region of the brain they are in becomes overloaded and impacts the section of the brain it is associated with, such as emotions or the ability to move body parts. As this overload passes to more neurons, the result can lead to sections of the brain becoming inoperable. This is known as an electrical storm where the nerves cells are firing too quickly.

A way to understand the impact of damaged neurons for those who have never had a seizure is through a computer system. There are the times when the computer suddenly stops working for a moment and the screen goes blank. A few seconds later, everything seems to be working again, except there is missing data and information that had been typed just prior to the screen going blank. In a sense, the computer had a partial complex seizure where major functioning components shut down momentarily and the memory was impacted.

Chemical imbalances in the brain are often caused by physical changes in the body and what is consumed. Stress, hormones, aging, diet, and injury are the key causes of the changes that lead to imbalances. Often, it is difficult to determine what the proper balance is and how to maintain it. Changes in the body's chemistry can trigger seizures, and medications work to resolve the imbalance.

---

[2]   Provided by Dr. Krauss of Johns Hopkins Hospital.

Seizure Stages and Types

There are three stages to a seizure: preictal, ictal, and postictal. The preictal stage is when a person is cognitive of what is around them, yet they have an odd feeling, taste, premonition, déjà vu, or sudden motion with a hand or foot. As the seizure continues to spread over partial or all of the brain, it transfers into the ictal stage. At first, the person becomes quiet, motionless, and stares straight ahead. Then, depending how far the seizure spreads, the body may stiffen and shake, and breathing may stop temporarily. Some people are not able to hold urine, others may vomit, while others may chew, grind their teeth, or clap their hands.

The postictal stage starts when the brain resets, and the person begins to regain control. This may last a few minutes or take days to fully recover. Since I had temporal lobe seizures, my ability to speak would take several minutes to a few hours to return, and to fully assemble thoughts could take a few days. This differs from an associate with temporal lobe seizures. She is able to speak and fully function normally after forty-five minutes of a grand mal seizure.

When diagnosed with epilepsy in 1964, there were only two types of seizures at that time: petit mal and grand mal. Through medical research, according to the Epilepsy Foundation of America®, seizures have now been identified and categorized into three major groups[3]:

1. *Generalized onset seizures* affect both sides of the brain or groups of cells on both sides of the brain at the same time. This term was used before and still includes seizure types like *tonic-clonic*, *absence*, or *atonic*, to name a few.[4] There are two categories of symptoms:

---

[3] The EPILEPSY FOUNDATION OF AMERICA, and EPILEPSY FOUNDATION are federally registered trademarks of the Epilepsy Foundation of America, Inc. The information is from their website; https://www.epilepsy.com/learn/types-seizures.

[4] More information concerning the types of seizures may be found in Appendix C.

- Motor symptoms may include sustained rhythmical jerking movements (*clonic*), muscles becoming weak or limp (*atonic*), muscles becoming tense or rigid (*tonic*), brief muscle twitching (*myoclonus*), or epileptic spasms (body flexes and extends repeatedly).
- Nonmotor symptoms are usually called *absence seizures.* These can be typical or *atypical absence seizures* (staring spells). Absence seizures can also have brief twitches (*myoclonus*) that can affect a specific part of the body or just the eyelids.

2. *Focal onset seizure* has replaced the category of *partial seizures, because,* the term *focal* is more accurate when talking about where seizures begin. Focal seizures can start in one area or group of cells in one side of the brain. Focal onset seizures are categorized based on the person's level of awareness during the seizure. This includes:
   - *Focal onset aware seizures* occur when a person is awake and aware during a seizure. This used to be called a simple partial seizure. Motor symptoms may include jerking (*clonic*), muscles becoming limp or weak (*atonic*), tense or rigid muscles (*tonic*), brief muscle twitching (*myoclonus*), or epileptic spasms. There may also be automatisms or repeated automatic movements, like clapping or rubbing of hands, lip-smacking or chewing, or running.
   - *Focal onset impaired awareness seizures* occur when a person is confused or their awareness is affected in some way during a focal seizure. This used to be called a complex partial seizure.

3. *Unknown onset seizures.* When the beginning of a seizure is not known, it's now called an unknown onset seizure. A seizure could also be called an unknown onset if it's not witnessed or seen by anyone. An example is when a seizure happens at night or when a person lives alone. As more information is

learned, an unknown onset seizure may later be diagnosed as a focal or generalized seizure. Seizures and Senses

A person's five senses and responsiveness are affected by where a seizure begins. Some people have seizures that start in the occipital lobe, and their vision is impeded. If the nerves continue to become overly excited, the seizure spreads to other sections of the brain and affects their other senses and abilities. If seizures begin in the hippocampus, the memory is affected; often the seizure spreads to vision, speech, and hearing. The centers of speech and memory recover slowly and, although the person can talk, their ability to comprehend and remember takes more time to fully recover. They can be more fearful of what is happening around them, or they can no longer laugh and play. Their ability to recall or recognize words may interfere with reading skills.

When seizures involve only a few sections of the brain, a person's cognitive abilities may not be completely interrupted during a seizure. A young woman's speech was interrupted, and she was staring straight ahead. Her father, who was nearby, came over and started to talk to her quietly, reassuring her that she was safe and everything would be okay in a couple of minutes. A few minutes later, her abilities fully returned as her seizure stopped and her brain reset. She was still able to see and hear while her seizure was occurring, even though she could not move her body or eyes.

Section 2

Personal Experience

Chapter 2

My Seizure History (1963–1968)

I have learned more about what my parents and siblings experienced with my first seizure as I work with the parents of very young children with seizures. Watching an adult have a generalized tonic-clonic seizure can be terrifying for people who do not know what a seizure is, especially with someone they love. Seeing a child have a seizure is considerably more difficult and emotionally stressful. I was four years old when I had my first seizure.

First Seizure

It was not until years later that I learned more about the impact my seizures had on my parents and siblings. In 1963, I developed a high fever from influenza. It started during the night while I was asleep. I have no memory of what happened, so my sister Kathy wrote of her experience. She was eight years old at the time.

> I would like to tell you my experience with your first seizure. I had faked being sick that day, so I didn't have to go to school. Mom had to go to the grocery store. She left us alone but told me Mrs. Small was going to stop by and make sure we were alright. It was getting late in the morning. I decided I needed to check on you to be sure you were alright. You were not alright. You were on your hands and knees in your bed unable to move. You could look at me. I was scared, but with the instincts of the future

nurse I would become, I decided to check your temp. Needless to say, glass thermometers were the only way to go. I got the thermometer and begged you to open your mouth, which was clenched shut. Somehow you managed to open your mouth enough for me to slide the thermometer under your tongue. Your teeth clamped shut, glass and mercury went everywhere including the inside of your mouth. I thought I had killed you! I started screaming "Spit it out!! Spit it out!" I do not know how you did it, but you managed to spit it out. I went hysterical and went downstairs. I loved you and did not want you to die. Mom came through the door of the kitchen where she met me, still absolutely hysterical. I told her what I had done. She ran upstairs, got you, and left to take you to the hospital. As she left, she told me to call Dad and have him meet her at the hospital.

The three days you were in the hospital, I worried. I did not want you to hurt or be sick. When you came home, I made sure you took your "little pill" whether I asked if you had taken it or whether I witnessed you taking it. I never wanted you to be sick like that again. I did not want you to hurt like that again.

I never faked being sick, again. Nor have I ever put anything in a seizing patient's mouth, again.

Keep in mind that cell phones did not exist, and our mother knew she had to get me to the hospital immediately. Kathy could remember the phone number of where our father worked and made the call. When we arrived, I was unresponsive, and my body began to shake and become rigid. It was not until late afternoon that my fever broke, and I became semiconscious of what was happening around me. Although the fever had subsided and the seizure stopped, I was exhausted and slept for several hours. My parents feared the outcome, for no one knew what I would be like when I woke up. Many years later, my mother asked me if I remembered the first thing I said when

I woke up and regained consciousness. I had no recollection. She said she would never forget it. I looked at her and said, "Mommy, I'm hungry."

To understand why this statement was important is realizing what can happen to the brain during a very high fever. In some cases, a very high fever may lead to the brain overheating, causing lesions or scar tissue as the neurons become damaged. While at the hospital, my parents had been informed there could be some serious consequences to my mental abilities. No one knew what the outcome would be until the seizure stopped and my system recovered. I was in the hospital for three days, being monitored for mercury poisoning. Test showed that I did not ingest any of the mercury. And being in a kneeling position at the time, the broken pieces of glass and mercury fell from my mouth. My mother found the mercury later on the bed. Two weeks later, I was taken to a hospital specializing in epilepsy where an electroencephalogram (EEG) was performed.

First EEG

An EEG is a test where a series of wires are attached to one's head for monitoring the electrical impulses occurring within the brain. This enables the doctors to evaluate if someone has epilepsy, for they will be able to identify an area of the brain that has been damaged. The damage is to the neurons that essentially become overloaded through an electrical storm. The EEG is relatively simple and is typically completed within an hour. However, as I would learn through experience with surgery, there are situations where the test may be done continuously for several straight days.

As a four-year-old, I feared having a bunch of wires attached to my head, especially when I had no idea why it was happening. The technician and my mother left the room, expecting me to take a nap. To this day, I remember crying and shouting to my mother, "Do not leave me!" They both immediately came back into the room, and my mother assured me she was not going to leave me behind. Even as a four-year-old, I knew something terrible was happening. I could not understand what was happening and was frightened that whatever it was, I would be isolated from my parents, just like I was during the night while I was at the hospital a few weeks earlier. Finally, I was comforted she would not leave me behind, so I lay down and closed my eyes.

When the test was over, my mother and the technician returned to the room. Mom did not say anything, and I knew something was wrong when I saw her face. The technician had shown her the results of the EEG, and they found an area where there was an electrical storm occurring in my brain. I remember how quiet my mother was, and she did not smile like she usually did. In fact, she did not say a word during our entire ride home. She was in shock as her four-year-old son had just been diagnosed with epilepsy.

Epilepsy is a condition that was, and still is, very misunderstood. Often, people were labeled and treated as mentally ill or unstable. In several states, people with epilepsy were not allowed to get married or go to school. In many cases, the child was placed in a special education group with children with learning disabilities. The lack of knowledge about epilepsy and the social stigma of the time had a significant role in my mother's response to my diagnosis.

Medication

In 1963, there were few medications available for treating epileptic seizures; the two primary medications available were phenobarbital and Dilantin. Within a few days, I started taking phenobarbital, which essentially slowed my brain down. When asked a question, I seemed to be unresponsive. The question would be repeated several times before I would provide an answer. My rate of speech had significantly slowed. My siblings referred to me as the old man because I acted like someone who was very old.

Personality Change

I was no longer the energetic little boy who laughed and cried and did silly things as young children typically do. I talked slower than a typical child, and my speech was impacted throughout my life due to medication. Fortunately, I was only on phenobarbital for four years. The doctors determined that an anticonvulsant was no longer needed. I had only the one seizure and had been seizure-free while on the medication, or so they thought. It would not be until years later when I learned the déjà vu and my visions of bugs in the house were *focal onset* seizures with nonmotor symptoms.

Family Impact

The impact on my family was in many ways typical. I was the youngest of four who required special attention during the child developmental years. My parents worried of what could happen. And this concern, although not expressed, was passed onto my siblings. My brother, who was the oldest, seemed to fade away. He later went into medical research and teaching, with a focus on children with birth defects. The younger of my two sisters, who tried to take my temperature while having the seizure, became an emergency room (ER) nurse and worked in this field for over thirty-five years. My oldest sister has applied her creative skills in illustration to medical text and training programs. The two of us have had a close relationship and grew even closer when she started having seizures. Initially diagnosed with epilepsy, she was eventually diagnosed with Meniere's disease. This is a condition that takes place in the inner ear, causing vertigo and loss of consciousness similar to seizures associated with epilepsy.

No Seizures

When I was eight years old, four years after being diagnosed with epilepsy, the doctors decided the seizures were no longer an issue, and I was taken off medication. A whole new me developed, and new opportunities came into my world. Scouting provided some wonderful camping experiences, sailing helped me learn what to do when the unexpected happened, and my father taught me about working with my hands and engineering.

I learned much from my father, who was an engineer, about engines as we serviced our cars and lawn mowers. He taught me how to replace sinks and fix leaky pipes, rewire electrical circuits, and work with the many tools as we did improvements to the old house we lived in. I learned about being creative and how there are many ways to solve a problem. When something broke, he would ask me what we should do to fix it. He would refine my solution to what was actually needed. He was teaching me about brainstorming, taking what comes to mind when facing a challenge, then refining it to resolve the problem. Some call this the engineer's manner of thinking.

When I was ten years old, I learned to sail a small boat on the Great South Bay, Long Island, New York. When I was fourteen, my parents bought me a Sunfish—a small fourteen-foot sailboat that enabled me to sail over to Fire Island. I loved sailing because it provided independence and emphasized the beauty and power of nature.

Great South Bay is a special place, for much of it is only two to four feet deep, and it is one of the largest clam beds in the world. I would sail for a while and then go to an area where I knew there would be clams buried in the sand. I would anchor the boat, step out into the shallow water, and find the hard shells of the clams by wiggling my feet into the sandy bottom. Upon feeling the hard shell of a clam, I would dive under, grab it with my hand, and drop it into the boat. Often I would sail back to the marina, store the boat, and ride my bike home with a bucket of clams hanging on the handlebars.

Through the Boy Scouts, I learned about camping, backpacking, and most importantly, leadership. I made Eagle Scout at the age of fifteen and did well in school. In 1976, I went with a group of scouts to Philmont, New Mexico, and backpacked 120 miles in some of the most beautiful country I had ever known. Just before graduating from high school and heading to college, I told my mother, "If I were to die today, it would be okay, for I have been able to achieve so much, and I've visited God's country."

Section 3

Student, Husband, Father (1977–2005)

Chapter 3

The University of Rhode Island

*I found two types of people: those who care about me
and those who fear me. With those who care, I found
a tighter bond. Those who feared me faded away. I
still felt a sense of rejection.*

When I graduated from high school, I went to the University of
Rhode Island where I majored in civil and environmental engineering.
Even though I did not know anyone at the university, I was excited to
be on my own, with an opportunity to earn a degree in engineering.
There were many students on campus who were willing to help the
new students get ready to start classes. During the first week, there
were events taking place to have people join one of the sports teams.
My passion for sailing took me straight to the sailing team, where I
quickly made new friends. I would crew for Brett and meet Bill, who
became an example for me on how to live with a disability.

The URI sailing team qualified for the Freshman Atlantic Coast
Championship at the US Merchant Marine Academy, Kings Point,
New York. The race was held on November 1977, with thirty-
three colleges participating. Each had two teams as the races were
separated into an A class and B class. Having the two classes enabled
the crews to have a break between races to rest and talk with the
coaches. Bill and another URI student were the A team; Brett and I
were the B team. The boats were rotated through the teams, because
any advantage to a particular boat would be for only one race, as it
would be rotated through the other teams.

The first day was a sailor's nightmare, as there was no wind. We
bobbed around the East River with an occasional light breeze and

completed three races when usually there would have been six to eight races.

Sailing Accident

The second day, the wind was blowing 20 mph with gusts over 30 mph, and the temperature had dropped to just above freezing with an occasional snow shower. This was a college sailors' dream for, at that stage of life, we were invincible.

During what would become the last race for the A team, we watched our teammates crash, or flip the boat over. As the tip of the mast hit the water, it bounced off the top of several waves. Bill and his crew managed to right the boat and complete the race. When they got back to the dock, Brett and I got in and sailed off. While we were waiting for the signal for start the next race, we noticed that the mast was tilted toward the back of the boat several inches. The forestay, or cable mounted to the front of the boat and held the mast in place, was pulled so hard when the A team crashed that it stretched and became longer. At the moment, we did not think this to be an issue because we were freezing from the cold weather. We had no warm gloves and did not wear much under our foul weather gear for it would get in the way. We were also busy and tired from hiking out that required leaning our body weight over the opposite side of the sail to counter the force of the wind and keep the boat upright.

The races started with the boats underway, and we maneuvered our boat to be in the best position as a horn sounded the start. We were no longer concerned about the cold for we worked so hard that we dripped with sweat like it was eighty degrees outside. We rounded the first mark in first place and took off like lightning for the second. Brett and I were now on a reach with the wind coming across the back of the starboard side of the boat. This required both of us to get as far back as possible to keep the bow of the boat from plowing into the water and flipping the boat end for end. As we came to the second mark, we both knew we were in trouble. When we were headed into the wind, we sat on one side toward the front of the boat. As we rounded the first mark, we were going downwind and had to shift our weight toward the back of the boat. Now with the mast tilted back, the boom came very low and into the back of the boat where we were. It could have easily hit us as it flew around to the other side as we changed direction. To make the turn around the mark, we had to jibe, which required changing direction with the wind coming from behind the boat and the power of the wind never leaving sail. Everything had to be timed perfectly.

Brett was sitting up on the back edge of the boat, and I was on the far back near the bottom of the cockpit. He pulled the helm over. And as he leaned back to get out of the way of the boom, he fell off the boat. His hand was so cold he could not let go of the tiller, and it caused the rudder to break off. I lay as low as possible. But as the boom came around, it slammed into the side of my head, bounced up, and hit the water on the other side of the boat. The boat toppled over, and I was thrown into the rigging. Within seconds, the boat was completely upside down.

I do not remember the boat flipping over and plunging into the water. When I regained consciousness, I was not able to move my body, but I could feel my legs. I was tangled in some lines, and Brett was pulling on the back of my foul weather gear. He yanked me out of the rigging and around to the back of the boat. He screamed, "Grab onto the rudder mount!" This was at the back of the boat where the rudder used to be. He hollered, but I could not hear him. Everything was in slow motion. The waves kept bashing us into the back of the boat, and he could not hang on.

I wanted to say something, yet the words were just not there. Eventually, my ability to hear and comprehend came back. Brett was holding onto me and the hull of the boat as best he could. Once he realized I could comprehend what he said and react appropriately, he got us on opposite sides of the boat so we could straddle the bottom by holding on to each other.

We did not know if we would be rescued in time. We were freezing and drifting very close to the Throgs Neck Bridge. As we lay there waiting for help, I saw my wool hat floating away. It was a very thick wool hat that kept my head warm and unknowingly cushioned the blow to my head. We had been washed off the boat hull by a wave. As the boat came down into the swell of another wave, we grabbed hold of each other and lifted partly out of the water as the boat was raised to the top of the next wave. We were tired, extremely cold, and struggled to hang on. When my ability to speak returned, I looked Brett in the eyes and calmly said, "I lost my hat."

For the next several years, the first thing Brett would tell people I introduced him to was "We were about to drown, and all Jon was concerned about was losing his hat." I was sad to lose it, for I knew the hat had saved my life.

After thirty minutes, we were picked up by one of the powerboats overseeing the race, and we were brought in. I was freezing, was shaking uncontrollably, and was quite blue. The left arm of my foul weather jacket was missing, and the left leg of my pants had been ripped off. I was so cold my genitals had completely retracted into my body, and I feared for a moment they were torn away too. This was probably exacerbated by the impact to my reasoning skills and cognitive abilities from the blow to the head. I was immediately taken to the showers where the warm water helped me regain my body temperature. I was relieved, as my genitals reappeared within a few minutes of being in the warm water. I was a man again.

I saw the boat when it was brought in and was amazed at the amount of damage that occurred; it was destroyed. The hull was cracked from one end to the other, the rigging was broken, the jib was ripped in two, and the main sail was torn. The boom was badly dented and warped where it hit my head. The rudder was never found.

During this time, I was not aware of the huge knot and swelling on the left side of my head. The coach looked me over and asked if I would be okay for the two-hour ride back to the campus. I assured him that I would be fine. We climbed into the car, and I fell asleep. I would soon regret not seeking medical attention.

No one realized the damage I suffered to my brain until the next day. The day after the accident, I had to take a history exam that involved writing essays. I had most of the facts; however, the paragraphs and sentences were incomplete. I had started a sentence but never finished it. Within a few weeks, I was having odd feelings in my stomach, and my hands would shake. Eleven months later, I had a grand mal seizure.

First Grand Mal Seizure

After recovering from the head injury, I had periods of high anxiety, my heart raced, and I felt a nauseous feeling in my stomach. The nausea would grow in intensity for a minute or two and then stop. I thought the anxiety was associated with my classes and assignments. Although I did not lose consciousness, I was experiencing a local seizure; my ignorance prevented me from seeking appropriate care.

It was early October 1978, my sophomore year, and I was determined on getting a 4.0 or perfect grades for the semester. It was a Friday afternoon, and there were approximately three hundred of us in a lecture hall, taking an exam for dynamics class. We had one hour to complete four questions. I was very tense. I could not sleep the night before and walked around the campus at 3:00 A.M. At breakfast, I ate very little because I could not chew the food without feeling as if I was going to vomit. At lunch, I drank some soup from the bowl for my hand shook so much I could not use a spoon.

In the lecture hall, I sat in the front row of one of the balcony sections and could see everyone in the class. There were four problems. And as I read through each one, my anxiety increased to a state where my mind went blank. Eventually, I could remember the equations and apply them to solve three of the questions. The remaining was the Ferris wheel problem; that required evaluating the forces people experienced at various stages of the ride. This was when I lost consciousness, and the grand mal seizure took over.

During the evening prior to the exam, I was experiencing the preictal stage of a seizure. The tenseness of my body, high anxiety, inability to eat, and feelings in my chest and stomach were similar

31

to a wave of nausea. The ictal stage came as the seizure spread and affected my eyesight. Peripheral vision was lost, and the only thing visible was the exam paper. As I stood up and screamed, the exam documents seemed to float away, and suddenly everything went dark. My classmates were shocked as they watched me stand up and scream and fall between the rows of seats and students. Those near me were stunned as I vomited, and my body shook uncontrollably.

My tongue was clenched between my teeth, and blood was flowing out of my mouth. A fellow student grabbed a small notebook and popped my jaw open so he could slip the book between my teeth. He knew how to do this because his father had epilepsy. Someone called the paramedics. Within ten minutes, I was rushed to the infirmary.

When I regained consciousness, the first thing I wanted to do was to complete my exam. I now knew how to solve the problem of the Ferris wheel—the one I could not remember how to do prior to the seizure. The craziness that had been ongoing in my brain was gone, and I could recall the equations necessary to solve the problem. The doctor called the professor and told me the professor was waiting to see me when I was ready to leave. When the doctor learned of my history of seizures, with this being my first in fifteen years, he changed his treatment plan. I was not allowed to leave, and he called my parents to inform them of what happened. They were told to come immediately to get me and seek appropriate medical attention.

My mother received the call at home then immediately called my father, who was closer to the campus due to where he worked in Garden City, New York. He had a calm disposition and was always one of the last to leave the building where he worked; however, this was the first time his staff saw him quickly tell an associate his son had a seizure as he ran out of the building. He set a record driving the 165 miles to the campus to see me. I felt totally exhausted, and I slept until he arrived.

My dad smiled at me as he walked into my examination room, and I could hear the doctor telling him what happened. He was pleased to see I was able to talk and stand on my own. I was still wearing the shirt covered in vomit, so in lieu of heading straight home, we walked over to my dormitory room where I could shower and change my clothes. We were soon on our way back home. This time, my dad drove within the speed limit. During the four-hour ride, we talked about what I could remember happening prior to and after the seizure. I had a splitting headache and felt exhausted; I slept for most of the ride.

Mom heard the car come into the driveway and ran outside to help me get out of the car. She looked very worried and was afraid of what happened. She was having flashbacks of witnessing me have the seizure when I was four years old. While she waited, she called her friends who were doctors and arranged for me to see a neurologist first thing Monday morning.

When I met the neurologist, I was told the seizure was nothing to worry about and was probably just a very unusual occurrence. I was told not to drink alcohol and to be sure to take my medication. He prescribed Dilantin and had my blood level tested a few days later. The test was done every hour for eight hours to see how my body reacted to it.

This occurred prior to 1996, when the Health Insurance Portability and Accountability Act (HIPAA) was enacted, and the neurologist was required to report the incident to the New York State Department of Motor Vehicles. His recommendation was, I should not lose my license over this unusual occurrence. Three weeks later, I received the letter from the Motor Vehicle Agency, notifying me that my license was suspended for a year. I was extremely frustrated; I had just refurbished a car, and I now had to sell it. I called the agency and requested an explanation as to why the license was suspended when the doctor did not recommend it. I was told this was state policy and there were no exceptions. I slammed the phone down and could not believe how rigid the agency was to people of my condition, especially when such rules did not exist for people dealing with other serious conditions associated with heart attacks or strokes. After reviewing the situation with an attorney, it was decided legal action would take longer than a year, so I agreed to wait it out.

Sail On

I never did give up sailing. In my junior year, I moved into a beach house near the university with my friends from the sailing team and continued to crew for Brett. The Windsurfer had just come out, and some people kept theirs at our house. I quickly learned how to sail a Windsurfer, and I loved it. Sailing taught me much about survival and to put my trust in God's hands. I found peace as I was sailing, powered by a force we cannot see and can change at any time. There was a similarity in this with my brain and seizures. Most of the time, sailing is fun. It is when the storms come that you need to be in a safe place. Seizures were the storms that occurred in my brain and can come at any time. With sailing and seizures, I cannot always be in a safe place when the storms occur.

Second Seizure

Five months later, during spring break, my friends and I went sailing in Florida. We had fun. I had no problems with seizures, and no one was concerned. In fact, I decided taking my medication was optional—to take only when I felt a need to. On this trip, I felt great and took little medication. We had been back on campus for less than a day when classes started. I made it through my 8:00 AM class and then went to a small auditorium where I was taking psychology. I found a seat and suddenly felt extremely tense. The nausea sensation came just a few minutes after I sat down and grew in intensity. My arms became weak, and I was losing parts of my vision. I looked at the person sitting next to me and calmly told her, "Goodbye." I have no memory beyond this point; however, my high school girlfriend was in the class and witnessed everything. She even rode in the ambulance with me to the infirmary. This time, I did not vomit, nor did I stand up and scream as had happened with the previous seizure. I went rigid for a few minutes and chewed/swallowed in a rhythmic fashion. When it ended, I was in a comatose form of sleep and did not know what happened until I woke up a few hours later. Even then, I could not tell the doctor my name or where I was. The doctor recognized me from my previous seizure and called my parents. My dad was quickly on his way to pick me up and take me home.

Basic Rules

This time I saw a different neurologist, and the visit had an impact on my accepting the diagnosis of epilepsy. Just as my mother and I were called into the doctor's office, he received an emergency phone call. For the next ten minutes, I sat there watching him talk on the phone to a woman who was crying for his help. She called from an emergency room where her husband was dying from a brain tumor. The neurologist kept telling her, "There is nothing else I can do for your husband. He is going to die." When he hung up the phone, he looked pale and talked to me very sternly. He started with "Jon, you have epilepsy." He knew I was not accepting my situation, so he gave me the five basic rules in controlling my seizures. These include the following:

1. Eat appropriately and don't skip meals.
2. Get eight hours of sleep, minimum.
3. Keep yourself hydrated—no alcohol.
4. Stay physically active; don't overstress, and be careful when you travel.
5. Take your medication.

He went on to say, "If you break one of the rules, you increase the probability of having a seizure. If you break two of the rules, you will probably have a seizure. If you break three of the rules, you will have a seizure. If you break any rule consistently, you will have a seizure!"

The most important was taking my medication; if I broke this one consistently, I could count on having a seizure. He then told me not to drink alcohol; however, being in college, he recognized I probably

35

would, so he gave me some basic rules about alcohol and medication: don't take both at the same time. Later, I conceded and stopped drinking alcohol altogether. When I went to the bars with my friends, I was getting my soft drinks for free. I took on the role of being the sober one of the group to make sure everyone got home safely. The tough part was, the clock started over on getting my driver's license reinstated. It would take another twelve months before consideration would be given by the Department of Motor Vehicles.

I had missed a week of classes, including an exam, and had a lot of work to make up. The toughest part was the fear now implanted in me concerning having another seizure. Would my ability to drive be revoked forever? Could I ever take another exam without my mind going blank and having another seizure? Would I ever be able to become an engineer? Depression set in as I struggled with the fear and consequences of seizures. I started asking the question "Why is this happening to me?"

A few days after returning to campus, my father sent me a letter addressing what he witnessed in me from the time he picked me up to dropping me off at campus a week later. He provided some guidance in dealing with tough situations, like the one I was in. In some ways, he could reflect on what I was going through for at the age of twelve, he was in a bicycle accident and nearly died from a head injury. His father had been notified by the police and was told to bring a pastor to the hospital to do the last rights. My father beat the odds and fully recovered. He wrote this:

> Dear Jon,
> When you left this morning, I felt you left quite reluctantly. This is quite understandable for home and parents represent a certain security that we all need . . .
> One of the key things in life that all of us must learn is that nothing is stable, everything changes. Some of the changes are for our betterment, some are not. The thing we must learn to do is adjust quickly to the

situation, good or bad. Nothing is ever all good or all bad so if we want to be happy then we must find the good in all situations and concentrate on it. Otherwise one can become very bitter and/or disillusioned.

In the case of your seizures you no doubt have said to yourself, "Why me?" All I can say is "Who knows?" The Bible says the sun shines and the rain falls on the good and evil alike. All the evidence says this has to be the answer to the question, "Why me?" Instead of worrying and being torn apart by, "Why me?" we have a better choice. That choice is "oh there is an obstacle in my path; how can I get around it, over it, under it, or through it? I will not give up my goals. If I have to modify the goals "OK" but as little as possible because I will get where I want to go . . .

All I want for you, Jon, is the good life and the only way I know to have the good life is to go forward. Sure, there will be setbacks and disappointments, but when they occur find a way to make up for what was lost and find the courage and drive to go forward again. If you do this I'm quite sure you will have a happy and full life.

Love,
Dad

I was relieved. I no longer felt I had to meet a standard *I* thought my parents wanted and I could not live up to. A perfect class average of a 4.0 GPA was no longer necessary. Most importantly, I was reminded how much my father loved me. He was my foundation for living through such difficult times. He inspired hope.

The day came when we were at a party and all my friends had too much to drink. Due to my medication, I had not been drinking, so it made sense for me to drive everyone home. Just as we were approaching a friend's house, the blue lights of a patrol car started flashing behind me, and we were pulled over by the police. When asked for my license, I told the officer I did not have one and I was driving because everyone else was intoxicated.

The officer did not believe me and had everyone get out of the car. With their adrenaline running, all but one of my friends could stand straight. The officer walked back to his car and radioed in the event to the dispatcher. While he was sitting in his car, the owner of our vehicle walked over to him and argued that I was telling the truth. I guess the beer on the fellow's breath, and the officer being trapped in his seat, convinced the officer that the people in the car were indeed unfit to drive. The officer realized what we had done was in the best interest of everyone.

When the officer was finished with the call in, he came over to me and apologized for not taking me seriously. He felt bad, for he had already called in the event to the station and could not cancel it. However, he was able to change the charge from "driving without a license" to "driving without a license on my person." At once my fear of being heavily fined and having a police record diminished. I just had to pay the state a twenty-five-dollar fine. The owner of the car got charged for the taillights not working. The officer directed me to never to do this again. He then told me to be safe and to drive everyone home.

Disabled

I did well with seizures for the next year, although I still had minor auras that today are considered simple focal seizures because I never lost consciousness. There were several people in my classes who no longer would associate with me for fear of my seizures. I was dealing with depression over what was happening in my life.

The person who kept me motivated was my friend Bill. Although he could not run well, he is a great sailor. In a race, he usually finishes in the top three. If he could live so well with it, I could live with the seizures.

My one-year driving suspension was over the end of my junior year. I got my driver's license back and felt like a free man again. My license was from New York, and I was now living in Rhode Island, so I talked to the staff at a satellite office of the local motor vehicle department. I was told there was no requirement for a doctor's certification every year as required in New York. I filled out the forms, answered the questions, and marked yes under diagnosed with epilepsy. I did not report that I had been given a ticket the year before. I was given my license and felt relieved.

Three months later, I was enjoying the beginning of my senior year when I received a letter from the Rhode Island Department of Transportation. They informed me that my license was suspended and tags revoked for lack of medical validation from my doctor that I was safe to drive. I felt like I was broken in half. I drove to the main office in Providence, Rhode Island, and met with the director of the motor vehicle department. He apologized for the misinformation by the satellite office and said there was nothing else he could do. He was going to delay any issuance of a license until a letter was received from my doctor validating my ability to drive based on my failure to report having a ticket for driving without a license the year before.

Suicidal Ideations

When I left his office, I sat down on a chair in the waiting area and was overwhelmed with a sense of desperation and hopelessness. I started to have thoughts of what I should do to get them to listen to me. The answer hit me immediately; all I had to do was to cut my wrist. The next thing in my mind was "I wish I had a knife." As soon as I had this thought, I heard another voice in my mind scream out *no*. It was like a slap in the face that brought me back to consciousness—the realization that if I were to follow that route of punishing those who hurt me, it meant being totally defeated by the system. That was not going to happen. I now had a challenge: learn to survive such dark times.

The following weekend, I hitchhiked to New London, Connecticut, where I rode the ferry to Orient Point on Long Island. From there, I hitchhiked to my parents' house in Bay Shore, New York. I was upset and needed someone to listen to me. My dad told me about the discrimination people diagnosed with epilepsy faced, especially with employment. He said, "If you want to work as an engineer, you cannot tell anyone about your seizures." He drove me back to the university that Sunday.

A few days after returning to college, I was waiting for a ride home at the entrance to the university. I was feeling sorry for myself and was very angry. At the entrance to the University of Rhode Island is the Rhode Island state seal. As I was looking at it, I had an epiphany—that moment in my life changed my perspective of everything that was happening. At the top of the state seal is the word *hope* with the symbol of an anchor below it. As long as I had an ounce of hope anchored in me, I could get through anything. It gave me a sense of God never giving up on me, and I should never give up on him. I had discovered the source of the "courage and the drive" my dad had written about.

Contact with an Angel

When the appropriate documents had arrived from my neurologist, my driver's license was reinstated. As I walked into the room where the car plates were distributed, I noticed there was no one else in the room, except the receptionist. As I approached him, he said, "I recognize you" (even though we had never seen each other and I had not introduced myself). He smiled at me and said, "I have something special for you." He was gone for a few minutes and came back with a license plate with my initials on it. When the story of my situation got around the agency, he took the time to order a special set of plates for me. All that had happened didn't sink in until a few days later. I wondered if he worked there, for his action was beyond anything I ever expected. Maybe this was a simple act of kindness by a state employee. Then again, maybe he was an angel looking out for me, or both.

Seizures and Sailing

In the summers between classes, I lived with my parents. To help pay for some of my college expenses, I got a job as a groundskeeper on an estate where I could keep my boat and continue to sail on Great South Bay. Eventually, I owned a Flying Junior—a two-person sailboat that was rigged for racing with a mainsail, a jib, and a spinnaker. This taught me a lot about how a boat reacts to an adjustment to the sail trim or other parts of the boat like the centerboard, which could be raised or lowered by adjusting one of the lines. With an oversized spinnaker, the boat would nearly come out of the water as it flew downwind. The spinnaker taught me about pushing my limits, as often the boat seemed to be on the verge of flipping over. Although it was designed for two people, I often went out by myself.

There were times I did lose control and the boat crashed. It was a moment when everything seemed out of control—a time when I had to gain control of myself to regain control of the situation. With the boat laying on its side and the sails in the water, I had to find the resources available to help in righting it or getting it upright. Although the wind knocked the boat over, it was the tool to lift it up again. The key was to point the mast toward the wind; I would then climb onto the centerboard and feel the boat start to come upright. As the mast came out of the water, the wind would blow under the sails and push the boat upright.

Similar to any challenging life event, I had to climb back on board and do an immediate assessment. The sails had to be cleared, the lines separated, and the water bailed out. The sails would flap in the wind, making lots of noise, and the lines used to trim the sails would flap around and cause the blocks to bang against the deck. Knowing how to sail and where everything had to be made recovery easier. Within a few minutes, I would be underway again, doing an assessment of what happened and what I learned from it, not only about the boat but also about myself. Later, when I started having seizures, sailing became a challenge as I learned to deal with the fear of seizures. Many times I had an aura while under sail, yet sailing had established a strong sense of self-confidence that enabled me to overcome the fear.

Many times, I had an aura (preictal stage of a seizure) while sailing and often feared getting on the boat. Once I was sailing, my fears abated for I had to pay attention to the boat and the wind. I could not see the wind; however, I could feel it, and I sensed the power as it made ripples on the water and powered the boat. It was a power I cannot control—only truly respect. I feel closest to God in such times. The government could make me stop driving but could not stop me from sailing. Sailing gave me an inner strength to face reality and ingrained confidence in myself.

The people I did not consider throughout all this were my parents. They let me continue to take the boat out even though they feared what would happen if I had a seizure while sailing, especially alone. Years later, my mom told my sister Susan how she would be filled with worry as I left the house until I returned. My parents never said I could not sail because they knew it was my manner of proving to myself I could still be me.

Things were looking up as I earned my bachelor's degree in civil and environmental engineering. I made dean's list several times, and people who got to know me learned why I talked slowly. It was not because of low intelligence, as many first assumed, but because of the damage to my brain and the effects of the medication I was on. My abilities were tested several times. I did very well in the courses that centered on mathematics and sciences. The hardest were the ones that required memorization and extensive writing.

After several job interviews, I was offered a job with the Navy at the Naval Base in Charleston, South Carolina. Through a friend I knew from the sailing team, I met several nurses who were officers in the Navy. If I needed any support, I had a group of people who could help me. This was important for after a few months of living in South Carolina, I had to have my wisdom teeth extracted. The nurses provided transportation and offered a place for me to stay for a few days if there were any complications. For several days, I could not eat any solid foods due to the pain in my teeth. I got a ride to the oral surgeon's office from an associate and proceeded with having all four wisdom teeth extracted.

One of the nurses, Suzanne, came to pick me up when the surgery was complete. When the technician came in to wake me up, she said, "Mr. Sadler [repeatedly], your wife is here to pick you up." As I sat up in the recovery room, I was dazed and bewildered—dazed by the anesthesia and bewildered on how I got married when I came in for a tooth extraction. Suzanne told me later how she got the doctor to change his prescription for the pain medication. She told him that what he initially prescribed and gave her to be filled increased the probability of my having a seizure. She laughed when I told her she was my wife.

Overstressed

The wisdom teeth pain and surgery played a significant role in my next seizure. I pushed my luck. It had only been two weeks since my wisdom teeth extraction when I decided I should go windsurfing in the ocean near where some of my friends lived. For nearly two weeks, I had been breaking the rules my neurologist told me concerning seizure triggers. I had not been eating or sleeping properly due to the pain in my mouth prior to and after surgery. The pain affected my sleep and minimized physical activity. I was tired, out of shape, and mentally stressed from the surgery.

My parents had come for a visit from New York and were on the beach with some of my friends and work associates. They were excited to be with me, meet some of my new friends, and see where I was living. I figured going windsurfing for a little while would assure them I was doing well and would not worry about me. They dropped me off at the end of the island, and I would sail to where they would be enjoying the beach several miles away.

The wind was blowing off the beach, so the ocean was calm. And I did not have to endure riding up the waves. I was a quarter of a mile from the beach and a couple of miles away from everyone when I realized how out of shape my body was as my arms and legs started to hurt from holding the sail in place. This was when the aura started. I tried to stop it by concentrating on sailing and adjusting the sail to relieve the stress in my arms. The aura kept getting stronger, and my arms were getting weaker. Eventually, I lost my balance, let go of the sail, and stepped into the water. It seemed that I was stepping off the edge of a cliff in slow motion. I could see, but my body would not react. I had no life jacket on, so I just kept sinking.

The thought of how my arms and legs should be moving to propel me through the water quickly passed as my body seemed turned off with no need to respond to what was happening. I could see, but I could not feel my hands drifting out in front of me, as if they were separate from my body. In lieu of being scared, I felt a total sense of peace as my body was suspended in the water, drifting down where there was no sound or fear, surrounded in tranquility. I was a third person, physically standing behind and looking through the window of my eyes in wonder of the water and the light. The water was getting darker as I sank deeper, and yet felt I was in a calm place and was not alone. I was in perfect peace as I thought, *So this is what it is like to die.*

Contact through the Soul

That was when I heard a calm voice say, "Not yet, Jon. I have plans for you." I immediately regained my old state of consciousness, and my mind and body came alive. The third person state of mind vanished, and I instantly started swimming toward the light and the surface. My lungs felt like they were going to burst, for I had not taken a deep breath when I stepped into the water and had not been breathing for some time. I battled not to breathe until I broke the surface, which seemed far away. I struggled to control my breathing as the panic alarm was going off in my head, and the natural instinct to breathe took over. I could not stop myself and started to exhale while still underwater. I swam faster and broke the surface just before starting to inhale. My chest felt like someone had severely beaten on it as I breathed rapidly. I had no strength and struggled to swim.

My Windsurfer was gone, and panic set in. Did it drift or sail away? When I turned my head, I caught a glimpse of it out of the corner of my eye. It was right behind me, less than an arm's length away. I grabbed hold and hung on until I could catch my breath. Feeling exhausted, I struggled to pull myself onboard and lay on the board while I regained some strength and orientation.

Eventually, I could stand, and I tried to pull the sail out of the water. It felt like a heavy log, but it eventually came upright. It took several more minutes before I could get underway. My eyes would not focus as I looked around me. The shore appeared to be a light-brown blur; the upper part of the sail would be there then disappeared. Where I needed to go was still far away. I was running very low on energy, yet knew I could make it, for the voice inferred there was much more in store for me. With time my vision fully returned and I could clearly see the shore. It seemed so far away that it should be impossible to sail in.

Fortunately, there were no waves that day and as I sailed up to the beach I fell off the board and crawled onto the dry land. My body was totally exhausted, there was nothing left. I was several hundred yards from where my parents were and could not get up to walk to them. I totally collapsed and lay face down in the sand.

Seems moms have a sixth sense. As my mom saw me coming onto the beach, she knew something was wrong and started running toward me. One of my housemates saw her take off and quickly followed. Here was a fifty-five-year-old woman outrunning a twenty-year-old college football player.

She knelt down next to me and asked what happened. I must have looked terrible, pale and unable to stand up. I told her I did not feel well, and asked my buddy if he could carry the windsurfer for me. My mom knew something else was wrong for I had trouble talking. Eventually, I had enough strength to stand and walk back to the group. I slept on the beach for a while and then walked back to the house. That night, when I told my parents what had happened; my mother told me she already knew, for she had seen this before. I did not say anything about the voice I heard until years later.

The neurologist was right. I broke more than three of the rules and had a seizure. Surgery, eating, sleeping, and dehydration were not taken care of—a primary setup for a seizure. The extent of the seizure was different from a grand mal, for I seemed to have some consciousness of what was happening but lost motor control (focal or partial seizure). Fortunately, I did not try to breathe while underwater.

Mark, the person I worked with and who had seizures, and I eventually rented a house on the Isle of Palms because of our love of the beach and boating. We had the best bachelor pad as he had two powerboats we could water-ski behind and explore the waterways and islands. I bought a used sixteen-foot Hobie Cat—a small twin hull sailboat that we kept on the beach. I would take the Hobie out by myself on days of moderate wind, and Mark would go with me when it was blowing hard. On our second time out, we achieved our summer goal of coming off the top of a wave and have the boat become completely airborne.

We loved to water-ski and pushed ourselves physically. We had fun living near the beach and working for the Navy. We stayed within the realms of the guidance provided by the neurologist as we ate well, stayed hydrated, and made sure we took our medications. We understood the importance of sleep and got a La-Z-Boy chair to promote taking naps. Playing hard was an important way of relieving stress.

I never gave up windsurfing and in fact have had much fun with it. One evening I went down to the end of Sullivan's Island and went windsurfing in the harbor. It was a beautiful evening, warm and clear. The tide was coming in, the flow was getting stronger, and the wind became calmer. As I pointed the Windsurfer back toward the island,

I realized the wind was not strong enough to overcome the tide. I was stuck, and for the next two hours I was carried farther away from my launch point.

There was a beautiful sunset, and the night set in. There was no moon, yet the harbor was lit with the light of the stars. I was surrounded by beauty yet frustrated that I could not sail home. Suddenly, the water lit up all around me as some creature circled around me and set off the photosynthesis of the plankton. For a moment I thought I was about to be devoured when I heard the blowing sound of the dolphins swimming around me. They were checking on me to make sure I was okay. Within a few minutes, the wind filled in, and I sailed back to the island.

When I got home, I found out how much my friends cared about me as they chewed me out for not letting them know what I was doing. They were frantic as they saw my Windsurfer was gone and had contacted the coast guard and had the police send out a boat to find me. It felt good to be loved.

Chapter 4

Husband/Father (1984–2005)

The most difficult part of having a seizure was watching my son talk to the paramedics. I felt hopeless, for I had no control over the rest of my body.

I met the person who became my wife through some friends who often came out to the beach to boat with us. She kept hearing, through her associates, about a fellow named Jon who lived at the beach and had all kinds of boats. We met at a group outing through work. She was intrigued by who I was, and we started dating. We fell in love and got married a year and a half after we met.

She was an officer in the Navy, so I came under the medical system of the US Navy. This started with filling out the paperwork for a Navy dependent to obtain registration and services. The form started with the officer's name and rank. For the spouse section, the form read "wife's name." I crossed this out and wrote *dependent* and then my name. At the time, the Navy was not ready for female officers with dependent spouses.

The Navy doctors were great. They reviewed my case history and saw that I had not had a seizure in nearly two years. They recommended, and I agreed, to be taken off medication. I was excited to be able to put epilepsy behind me. There would no longer be any issues with getting a driver's license or working as an engineer. I was going to be freed from effects of seizures and medications.

Our First Seizure

About a month later, I was to attend a work-related class held in the evening in downtown Charleston. I planned to drive downtown after eating dinner at home. I could not believe how anxious I was. For some reason, I was very worried about finding the place and being on time. This grew more intense, and I started to be concerned about how I would come across to the people I would meet, especially upper management. Over the next hour, my fear intensified, and I could not understand what was happening. The fear transformed into anxiety, and my hands began to tremble.

We had just moved into our new house, and I was sitting at the kitchen counter. The anxiety reached a point where I started to feel I could not move. Then the wave of nausea hit me as the aura started. I got up to get away from the counter and was trying to get to the couch twenty feet away. The aura continued to intensify, and I collapsed halfway to the couch onto the carpeted floor. My wife saw me hit the floor. My eyes were open but were not responding, and my face was distorted. I was chewing on my tongue, and blood was trickling out my mouth. When she tried to pull my mouth open to free my tongue, I unconsciously bit her, and now she required medical attention. She got up, ran to the phone, and called 911.

I do not remember biting her, but I do remember the paramedics arriving. I could hear them talking to my wife as they came into the room. They saw my body was a shade of blue from not breathing. They cut off my shirt, attached leads for a heart monitor, and gave me oxygen. I could not move, but I was aware of their work. They asked me simple questions such as "What is your name?" and "Where are you?" I could not respond. The question registered in my mind; the answer and the ability to speak was not there.

I was in a different world. I could see light but could not move my eyes or relate to what I could see. After several minutes of talking with my wife and observation, the paramedics recommended transporting me to a local hospital. I could comprehend yet not speak, so I shook my head no. A few minutes later, my speech began to return, and I signed a form stating I did not want to be transported. My wife agreed for we did not want to go to a local hospital with the confusion it would create with the Navy health care system.

When the paramedics left, I had no strength, so I continued to sit on the floor and leaned against the wall. My mind started to realize what had happened. I had lost all control of myself, and my wife saw the dark side of me. As reality was setting in, I lost control of my emotions and cried hard. My wife knelt down beside me and held me. She was scared too.

After about an hour, I got up. I was weak and sore all over. I washed the blood off my face and changed my clothes. My wife drove me to the Navy hospital where I was examined. An appointment was scheduled for the following day. The doctors seemed more interested in treating my wife, for the bite from a human can cause serious infections. She was given medication, and the wound was treated. As we drove home, I slipped into a deep state of depression, unknowing what was going to happen to me. I just knew I would lose my job and be restricted.

Navy Doctors

The first thing we did the following day was to see my doctor at the Navy hospital. His first comment was "Looks like we [referring to him] made a mistake."[5] I was placed back on medication (Dilantin), and my mouth was checked over again. I asked about being reported to the state motor vehicle department, losing my driver's license, and the restrictions in working in construction. I was assured I had nothing to worry about; the Navy did not come under the jurisdiction of the state. A thirty-day driving restriction was placed on me by the doctor to assure my medication was at an appropriate level to control my seizures. A letter was provided to give to my supervisor

---

[5]   Although I had been having auras at the time, no one correlated these as a form of seizure, for they had no impact to my cognitive abilities. This is now considered to be a focal onset aware seizure.

concerning my absence and driving restriction. As I prepared to leave the room, I was told not to push myself too hard for a couple of days to allow my body to recover.

My next stop was to see my supervisor at work. I explained the situation and provided the letter from the doctor. He was concerned about my welfare and assured me everything would be fine. He arranged for me not to drive and expressed his willingness to help in my recovery. Then he called the chief of the inspection team and had the inspectors help me continue what I typically did—visit construction sites. Psychologically, it was the best thing anyone could do for me. He did not want me to just sit in the office and isolate myself. I was exhausted yet relieved to know I could still be an engineer and continue to work. My wife gave me a ride home. I went to bed and fell into a deep sleep. She went back to her office.

I took another day off and then had the weekend to recover. On Monday, one of the inspectors took me with him to review some work he was overseeing. We stayed in the safer areas of the site— ground floor of a building— just in case I had another seizure. The work was nearly complete, and no equipment or hazards were present. We then drove by some sites where we could review the initial phases of construction from his vehicle. Things began to look promising as the people I worked with were concerned about me and willing to help. My fears of how others would respond to my seizures diminished, and my depression melted away.

Contract with God

As I was learning about construction contracts, I thought it would be a good time to make a contract with God. I told God that I would continue to do my best, with the skills I was blessed with, and be a good person to those I met if I could control my seizures for twenty years. He seemed to agree, and my seizures were controlled. For the next six years, everything was going extremely well with my relationships, employment, and physical and mental abilities. My weekends were spent on the water or at the beach with my wife and friends. I had terrific health care, and my supervisor was very supportive. I did not have to worry about losing my job if I had a seizure. Life was good!

When my wife completed her obligation with the Navy, she moved to Philadelphia to go to graduate school. I was to go to Mobile, Alabama, and be the resident engineer in charge of construction of a new naval station. Soon after she started graduate school, the Navy considered cancelling the Navy station in Mobile. After several months of waiting to know if the cancellation was going to happen, I decided to move to Philadelphia. I declined the offer to be the resident engineer and transferred to the northern division of the Naval Facilities Engineering Command in Philadelphia, Pennsylvania.

We were apart for four months until I could make the transfer. To stay busy, I planned on taking the Professional Engineer (PE) Exam for the third time (I failed by two points the first time and did not have time to study the second time). This time I was much better prepared with notebooks organized by subject with appropriate equations, tables, and example problems. My biggest fear was having no one with me if I had a seizure, the stress involved with exams being a key trigger. During the exam, I had several auras, yet I finished on time. A few months later, I learned I had passed and was very excited. This opened up many high-level positions within the Naval Facilities Engineering Command.

Seizures in Philadelphia

The stress of living alone was causing me to have more auras, and moving to Philadelphia, Pennsylvania, and changing jobs made the stress more intense. Within a few months of relocating, I was playing racquet ball with a friend. We waited for a court to become available at the indoor facilities on campus. The ventilation system was broken, and the court was hot and smelled poorly from people playing hard and sweating profusely. We had just started to play when I felt the aura come on. This time the nausea was more intense than usual as I could feel it in my arms too. My heart was racing. I told my friend I had to leave and ran out the door. I remember running off the court and starting to walk down a series of steps. The next thing I knew, I was back in my apartment.

My friend told me I seemed to be walking fine; however, I was babbling, and he could not understand me. As we came outside, I continued to walk straight onto the busy street. He grabbed my arm, pulled me back, and led me to his car. I did not know how to get in, so he opened the door and guided me in. I did not remember riding in the car or walking back to the apartment from where he parked a few blocks away. He struggled with being unsure if he should take me to an emergency room right away. Then he realized my wife would know what to do, so he drove back to the apartment complex we lived in. When we arrived, he guided me out of the car and up to my apartment.

My wife explained my epilepsy and thanked him for helping me. Her assurance that I would recover helped my friend calm down. He felt much better as he walked over to his apartment. I was exhausted and slept for several hours.

The following weekend, we played squash again—only this time there had not been anyone on the court before us, and the ventilation worked. I had no problems with seizures and felt I could continue to play the game. My friend was much relieved, too, especially when he won this time. We laughed as I told him I felt obligated to let him win. We played many more times together, and I never had another seizure during a game.

Baltimore, Maryland

When my wife finished her degree, we moved near Baltimore, Maryland, and shopped for a house. Within a year, we found a nice place to live. We were excited with our marriage, work, and new home. A few months after we moved in, we both got a case of the flu. Both of us had fevers and felt miserable. I had not been able to eat, drink, or take my medication for over a day.

My low-grade fever suddenly spiked, leading to two grand mal seizures in one day. When the auras started, I laid down on our new couch (the only piece of furniture we owned for our living room at the time). Both times as I came out of the seizure and regained some consciousness, I could see my wife close to me, watching what was happening. There was nothing she could do except help me take ibuprofen and hope the fever broke. Early that evening, the fever went away, and I did not have any more seizures. It would take several days for my mental abilities to fully recover as I had difficulty assembling words. I would start to say a sentence and not realize I never finished it.

Positive Attitude Dissolving

As long as I could figure out the cause of the seizures, I felt some control. New doctors, new medications, and more knowledge of what we were dealing with helped me keep a positive attitude. I had left civil service with the Navy and started working for a construction firm in Baltimore. This was very challenging and stressful as we had schedules and budgets to meet.

My sleep was often disrupted as our first child, Wesley, as a newborn, often affected my sleep. The stress associated with my new job was getting to me, leading to several minor seizures a week. The stress was further exacerbated by being dependent of a coworker for transportation.

With my seizures so out of control, my internal medicine doctor told me to go to Johns Hopkins Hospital to see if they could provide treatment to get my seizures under control. I was terrified, for this meant my seizures were so intense I now had to seek medical care from one of the leading epilepsy research facilities in the world. After the initial testing and evaluation, I was placed on several medications. Although they seemed to stop the seizures, the side effects severely affected my ability to mentally process information. This affected my family and work, and I decided it would be best to seek a second opinion. I started seeing another neurologist at a different hospital whose approach best fit my situation. I would see Dr. Krauss fourteen years later when my seizures became intractable.

Finding Proper Care

It was the spring of 1991 when I had my first visit to Dr. Johnson's office; my wife and Wesley were with me.[6] Wes was a few months old, and we carried him in a car seat / cradle. When we entered the doctor's office, Dr. Johnson had us put Wesley on the end of his desk. As I talked about the types of seizures we were dealing with, the doctor's eyes became more focused on Wesley, and he began to get pale; a deep expression of sadness came over his face. When I presented my history of seizures, he took his eyes off Wesley, breathed a sigh of relief, and said, "You're the one with epilepsy. I thought it was your child you were referring to. I can help you." I knew he would be the best for me for he was open and willing to work with me as an individual. He became my neurologist over the next twenty-five years.

Emotionally, I was torn apart. I feared losing my job and not being able to take care of Wesley. My wife had to go out of state for three days of training, Wesley was three months old, and I was going to be a single parent. As my wife was getting ready to leave, I took Wes for a walk. We were less than a block away from the house when I broke down. I was overwhelmed with the fear of having a seizure and could only imagine the worst outcomes. Soon after my wife left the house for her trip, I looked at Wes, and he smiled at me. This time my tears were filled with joy. The next three days were focused on him and not me, and I had no more thoughts or issues with epilepsy.

---

[6] To maintain privacy the doctor's name has been changed.

It seemed that every time I had breakthrough seizures, a new medication was available for me to try. Most worked very well for a couple of years. When I started having minor breakthrough seizures, my neurologist would prescribe a different medication. Dilantin was the baseline, the new medications secondary. When I had reactions either physically or mentally to a medication, there seemed to be another recently developed that minimized my seizures for a few more years.

Wesley became aware of and was concerned about my seizures at a very young age. Some of his earliest memories came from seeing me have a seizure. I kept trying to get him to say his name in case I had a seizure while away from home. He seemed to be very serious and did not say anything for over two years. In fact, we thought there was an issue with his mental development. One day we were outside eating dinner on our deck when a fly started pestering us. I tried to kill it by clapping my hands together as it flew in front of me. Some of Wesley's first words came as he said, "Uh oh, Daddy." He thought I was having a seizure, for I often clap my hands during the ictal stage. He could sense something was wrong.

Going sailing had a calming effect on me. To help manage my stress, I volunteered to crew on a thirty-four-foot sailboat in a regatta held every Wednesday evening in Annapolis, Maryland. Concentrating on sailing helped me keep everything else in the right perspective. The race would start at 6:00 PM and would be over in an hour or two, depending on how strong the wind was blowing. We would bring the boat in and have dinner consisting of some sandwiches and chips together.

One evening, there was very little wind, and we were late finishing. I was feeling tired and unusually anxious as we ate dinner together. As I was driving out of Annapolis, I saw the replicas of two of the ships Christopher Columbus sailed when he discovered America. My anxiety continued to build, and I could not figure out why. Driving down the highway, I could see the dark outline of the trees along the edge, and my anxiety continued to increase. Finally,

I felt the aura start as a wave of nausea flowed down my chest and into my stomach.

I debated on whether I should pull over or not. Usually the aura would soon go away. This time it lingered and started to increase in intensity. There was a car on the side of the road and someone taking a tire off it, so I pulled up several yards behind them and put my car in park. That was the last thing I remembered for the next several minutes.

My car was running the whole time, and the person thought I was working on something in my car. When I could see again, they were done and walking toward my car. I waved to them, hoping they would come help me. Apparently, they thought my wave was an indication I did not need assistance, so they turned around, walked back to their car, and drove away.

For several more minutes, I sat in the car, wondering why I couldn't see. I was confused, and everything was very blurry. I thought the seizure was continuing as my vision would be focused for a moment then immediately go blurry again. It took several more minutes for me to remember I wore contact lenses and the one in my dominant eye had fallen out during the seizure.

As my senses returned, my tongue hurt, and there was saliva and blood on my shirt. I covered my dominant eye so I could see to drive. The highway seemed very unfamiliar even though I had driven the route many times. I could not remember how to get home. Soon there was an exit ramp that looked familiar, and it took me onto the beltway around Baltimore. This was the exit I needed, but I wasn't sure, so I got off at the next exit. I was becoming lost.

After driving a while, I realized I needed to turn around and get back on the beltway. I managed to make a U-turn and was having trouble finding the access ramp onto the beltway. I wasn't familiar with the area, and my vision was blurred to the point I could not read the signage. Then there were some green signs associated with the highway, and I followed it. Suddenly, there was a ramp I recognized that brought me back on the beltway. I was fortunately going in the right direction. Twenty minutes later, my memory was coming back, and I knew how to get home.

It had been over an hour later than usual in my getting home. My wife was awake and wondering where I had been. I told her about the seizure—that I was scared and extremely tired. I told her to please contact her associate and let her know I could no longer crew for them. I changed my clothes and fell into bed. My head throbbed, and it would be a while before I fell asleep, even though I was exhausted.

Working for a general contractor was too stressing and taxing for my body and brain. Now with a child and my wife working in real estate and me in construction, we were concerned of losing our jobs if the market were to crash. I decided to return to civil service and work for the Army Corps of Engineers.

Two years later, we had our second child—Steven. Steve was much more laid back and seemed to rely on Wesley. As they grew older, I would hear Steven ask Wesley about my seizures. Steve seemed less intense yet just as concerned.

Dr. Johnson was very good at helping me regain control. It seemed whenever there was a breakthrough seizure, a new medication would have been approved for me to use as a secondary seizure control medication. He referred to me as the "Jaguar [car] we have to keep finely tuned or your system [brain] stops working."

Children, Driving, and Seizures

I refused to be isolated and stayed active with my children. Both liked to play sports, so I coached soccer and baseball teams when they were five to when they were ten years old. I had a lot of fun being with all the children on the teams. I learned a lot about leadership from the children, as I had to be able to associate with them at their level. It was an opportunity to teach my son Steven how not be afraid of people who were bigger than him.

Steven was five and had just started to play soccer. He would give the ball to the children who were bigger than him. There was one child on another team who was a head taller and twenty pounds heavier than Steve. Everyone would give the ball to this big kid because they feared what he may do.

One morning, we were in the kitchen and had a talk about why Steve would pass the ball to this boy. He told me he was scared of what bigger people could do to him, so we talked of the advantages smaller people had on big people. I explained our advantage was how we were closer to the ground and were tripping hazards to the big people. He didn't believe me until we did a little drill. He ran at me as I dramatically ran toward him. When he hit my legs, I went over the top of him and crashed to the floor. He quickly turned around, and his mouth dropped open in disbelief. So we did it again. I also taught him how to be the intimidator by screaming as he goes for the ball. We practiced many more times in the kitchen, laughing each time I wound up on the floor.

In the next game, the big kid had the ball and was coming down the field. Suddenly, Steve came running as fast as he could across the field and, as he came up to the ball, let loose with this loud shriek. The big kid looked up. And as he saw Steve coming at him, he stopped, and Steve tore the ball away from him. He never gave the ball up again, and some of the other children on the team started doing the same thing. The whole team did much better that year. It would take three more years to teach Steve not to scream as he came after the ball.

Steve and Wes got into scouting, so there were the various leadership positions for me to volunteer and new friends to be made along the way. I was feeling good and doing well at home and at work. I was confident I could maintain control of my seizures with the support of Dr. Johnson and the new medications that were becoming available about the time of any breakthrough seizures.

One summer, I took on the role of being the scoutmaster at summer camp with the younger boys. It was in July 2004 when Wes was thirteen and Steven was ten. For Steve, it was his first time going to summer camp with the scouts. The week went well; however, my sleep and eating were severely hindered. The food available was what was served at the dining facility, and it wasn't the best for me. Cleanliness was not the same as at home. On some evenings, we ate at our campsite where the boys prepared the food.

I was up late going to the adult leadership meetings after the boys went to bed. These were good meetings to share with other scoutmasters what to expect and review the schedules for the next day. Usually I was the first one up in the morning, getting less than five hours of sleep per night. They always say, "To be a scoutmaster takes one hour a week." (I would joke with friends of how the fine print said "one hour per week per boy.") To keep going, it seemed my system was running on adrenalin and was being physically stressed out.

On the morning of our last day, I overslept and was awakened by an aura. It did not seem bad, and I walked by myself to the bathroom. While there, I had another slightly more intense aura. The aura consisted of a wave of nausea that started slowly and intensified over a few minutes. I could feel and hear my heart race. When I looked in the mirror, I was very pale, yet I had not lost consciousness. I was left with a high level of anxiety that persisted and would not go away.

Later in the morning, we were packing up all our equipment and checking out. The boys had done extremely well, and I was proud of all of them. By late morning, everything was ready, and two of the parents arrived to take a group of the boys back to the church that sponsored the troop. There they would put the equipment away and their parents would meet them. I should have been able to let myself calm down for I was no longer responsible for all nine boys, yet the anxiety persisted. All we had to do was make a stop at the church, then home.

Although there were people who could help me, I did not feel I needed to ask. Here I had taken responsibility for their children all week, and we were so close to everything coming to closure. I thought I could drive home. On the way to the church, I had an aura while driving. This one wasn't nearly as bad as the last one, so I kept driving. We arrived at the church, and we unloaded the truck and made sure all the boys were picked up. Wes, Steve, and I were the last to leave, and I was still feeling anxious. We were only ten minutes from home now, so I figured I would be able to make it. I had had several auras without losing consciousness and thought my medication was working and was effective.

With everything unloaded at the church and all the boys returned to their parents, we headed for home. We were less than a mile and a half away when I felt another aura coming; this one was more intense than the others. We were so close to home I thought we would be able to get there before the seizure went critical, if it did at all. Just as we came through the entrance to the community we live in, I lost consciousness, and my foot went down on the gas pedal.

Wes had known something was wrong with me even though I had not said anything. He rode in the front passenger seat, and the moment I started to lose control, he was prepared. He took off his seat belt and climbed over the center console of our Chevy Avalanche while trying to keep control of the steering wheel. The truck went speeding down the hill and hit the curb several times. Steve was in the back seat and witnessed all of it.

A few seconds later, I regained some consciousness and was very confused. My vision was blurry, and I was looking down toward my feet. I had no sense of touch and could not feel anything through my hands and feet, but I was relieved to see my foot was on the brake and the truck was stopped. Suddenly, I saw a third foot near the driver's door. Whose could this be? Why was there another boot on the floor? As my vision cleared, the boot by the door and near the gas pedal was the same style and size. It would take a few more minutes before my peripheral vision would come back, and I could comprehend a leg attached to the third boot went up to my right. As I looked over that way, I could see Wesley. It was his boot pressing on the brake pedal. We were now less than a tenth of a mile from home.

Being so close to home, I told Wes to let off the brake and I would drive the rest of the way home. He was upset and asked if this was a smart thing to do. I assured him I could and was able to drive the rest of the way home. He sat beside me and kept his hand on the wheel. We pulled into the driveway and came to a stop.

My wife was at the house and could see something was wrong. I could not answer her questions for my speech was impaired by the seizure. Wes told her what happened as I went to bed and slept for several hours. It would take me several days to fully recover. My body hurt, and my tongue was sore from chewing on it. I was depressed and was beginning to realize the impact my seizures had on my children.

A few days later, while going to work, I could see the tire marks from my truck on the curb. We hit the curb five times at a speed over 50 mph. Had Wes not been able to knock my foot off the gas pedal and get enough pressure on the brake to bring us to a stop, we would have plowed into the trees at the end of the road, one block from where we stopped. In his position, struggling to get control of the truck, the engineer in me realized Wes would have had nothing keep him in the truck, except the windshield, if we hit a tree. A windshield is insufficient to protect someone when coming to a sudden stop while traveling at 50 mph. I thought for a long time how close Wes came to being seriously injured or killed and of my lack of acknowledging the impact my seizures had on my family and other people. I felt riddled with guilt and a sense of despair. There was no one available to me that I could talk to who would understand and be able to help me.

I had many auras throughout this time, and they were coming more often. Little did I know that with each seizure, more damage was occurring in my brain. Most of my left hippocampus was damaged and shut down, except for the firestorms that kept occurring in that area.

Breaking the Travel Rule

It was the spring of 2005, nearly a year after my seizure while driving, when we made a trip to visit friends and my wife's aunt in California, far from where we lived in Maryland. On the second day, we were at the aunt's farm, and I did not feel well and had no energy. It was a Sunday morning, and we went to church—an outdoor facility with lots of people. The anxiety attacks started as we were introduced to others. I did not feel comfortable around so many people and had difficulty responding when we were introduced. It seemed my brain was acting in slow motion and could not locate even some basic words.

When we returned to the farm, I went to bed and slept for a couple of hours. When I woke up, my tongue and the side of my mouth hurt from a seizure that occurred in my sleep, causing me to chew and drool. I felt exhausted yet obligated to be social, so I joined everyone for lunch. I didn't eat anything or say anything about the seizure. Everyone was excited about being on the farm, and the boys, my wife, and her aunt and uncle went outside. I was sitting on the couch, and my wife's 102-year-old grandmother was near me.

I was drifting in and out of sleep when I felt the aura come and rapidly intensify; a wave of nausea and high anxiety caused my body to tremble and heart to race. The seizure quickly magnified, and my body went rigid and shook. For a moment I could see total darkness as a battle was raging in my brain. Part of me was screaming for control while another part was cut off, in total darkness. My vision would flash on for a second and then cut off—back to the darkness and the void. When my vision was effective, I could see the grandmother (who was nearly blind) getting upset. She was shouting for help (I could not hear her), and there was no one there to help her. Her blindness prevented her from getting up and finding someone.

My body would go rigid for several seconds, then relax. My breathing was erratic. The uncle, who was just outside the house, heard the grandmother and came running into the room. When he realized what was happening, he went to his closet and grabbed his shotgun, which he kept handy to protect the animals on the farm. He ran outside and fired several times to get my wife's attention. She and the boys were out riding in the field on an all-wheel drive vehicle. My wife heard the gunfire and immediately headed to the house. I could see her come into the room, but I could not respond. I heard her immediately say, "Call 911." I could see the fear in my children's eyes.

My body turned blue from interrupted breathing, and I could not talk. My right leg hurt from having it under the couch where it could not go straight when the muscles seized. Some muscle in the thigh had been stretched and torn; there was a lot of pain. When the paramedics arrived, I was given oxygen, and started to recover. The blueness in my flesh quickly faded, and my color came back, although I was pale from exhaustion.

Transportation to the hospital was deemed necessary for blood test and observation. I needed to urinate, and although I could not say so, I was able to communicate with the word *bathroom* and point to it. I was provided assistance as I walked over and then given some privacy with the door partially opened so the paramedics could respond if I fell. The gurney had been transformed into a chair so I could be carried down the stairs. This was necessary for I could not comprehend how to go down the steps, especially with the injury to my leg. On the way to the hospital, the paramedic asked me numerous times, "What is your name?" and "Where are you now?" I could not answer him until shortly before getting to the hospital. Even then all I could say was "Jon" and "I am in an ambulance." It had been over an hour since I regained consciousness.

I felt like I had just been in a major fight as my head ached and my body was exhausted and hurt, not only in the leg but also throughout. My tongue had been clamped between my teeth, and the walls of my mouth were chewed on. It hurt to walk, and it took an effort to move my arms. At the hospital, blood tests were immediately performed, and the results indicated my medication level was very low. I had been taking my medication as scheduled; however, something with the travel to California and possibly having a twenty-four-hour flu impacted how fast it was metabolized.

My wife and I slept at our hotel that night while the boys stayed with her aunt and uncle. They were to stay with us at the hotel; however, we figured they would not sleep well being worried about their dad, especially when I had another seizure. I was concerned about my wife's grandmother and what she witnessed. Overall, I felt like crap—physically and emotionally—from what people witnessed.

Although I was very concerned about everyone, I fell asleep for my body was physically and emotionally exhausted.

The next day, we returned to the farm to check in and be with the boys. Wes did not appear to have slept much as he told me how worried he was about losing me. What he saw prior to the paramedics arriving had him thinking I was going to die, and there was nothing he could do. His younger brother, Steven, was trying to understand everything that happened. He hadn't slept well either. The grandmother was pleased I was back, and we talked for a while about what it was like for both of us. I told her I could see her while having the seizure and saw her yelling for help. I felt bad about what she was witnessing, even while having the seizure. I was assured everything would be okay and was reminded how I need to take care of myself. I was then told we were going to have a birthday celebration; I could not remember it was my forty-sixth birthday.

Depression Sets In

Something was happening within me, and my ability to live with seizures was diminishing. I had been on numerous medications and combinations thereof. Some had severe impact to my personality; others worked fine for a couple of years, then they stopped being effective as I had breakthrough seizures. I was very nervous every time I saw my neurologist for I feared there were no new medications available to control my seizures. I called him when we returned from California to talk about what happened and what we should do.

Soon after this, I slipped into a state of depression that lasted several days. It returned with the changes of the seasons. The most intense came in the fall, with the decrease in the amount of daylight, and lasted several weeks. Nothing seemed to be going right. I felt everything I owned and cared for would be lost as my seizures became intractable. Rejection by others was my greatest fear, enhanced by the limitations with transportation. Sometimes I felt like I had a gun to my head and someday it would go off.

I would take our golden retriever for a walk, and when I returned, I thought maybe it was time to die.[7] Was this me or a side effect of the high dose of medication required to keep my seizures under control? I did not know. All I knew was it was happening regularly, and it was staying with me for longer periods of time.

As I struggled through the next couple of years, I relied on a strong faith that was being tested. It must have been God telling me years before while windsurfing, "I have plans for you." If such plans really existed, what were they? I had been the project manager on a national monument to the Korean War veterans, which required all my knowledge and skills in construction. It was extremely challenging and touched thousands, so that must have been the plan. My twenty-year contract I made with God was up, too, yet I was still alive. There must be more than this, for my boys were in high school and middle school. I needed to be available for them.

No More Medications Available

In the spring of 2005, my neurologist told me there was a new medication called Lamictal that could be very effective for me. Due to the potential for side effects, I was to see him within six weeks for a follow up. When the appointment time came, I had numerous cold sores in my mouth and was directed to immediately stop taking the medication for such reactions were an indicator the medication may do serious damage to the body's organs. Phenobarbital was prescribed, which caused me to slip into a deep sleep, and I could not stay awake. I was basically nonfunctional. We had run out of medications to try; there was nothing else out there for me to treat my seizures. I would stay on Dilantin and hope something new would come along soon.

---

[7] Years later, while studying psychotherapy, I learned about suicidal premonitions/ideations. This is a time when someone has thoughts about suicide without a plan to carry it out.

More Seizures

Three months later, the fall season came. The daylight became shorter, and the stress associated with school starting for the boys and work obligations made me more susceptible to breakthrough seizures. I started having one to two simple partial seizures a week. After being on so many different medications and having breakthrough seizures, the seizures were now considered intractable. They were no longer controllable through medications. My brain was now damaged to the extent that even low-level stress and minor changes to diet and sleep triggered seizures. My doctors informed me I needed more extensive care as the epilepsy spun out of control.

Section 4

Professional Career

Chapter 5

The Navy (1981–1989)

The only thing you will ever be allowed to do is to sit
at a desk and sharpen pencils.

My career as an engineer started on June 30, 1981, with the Navy at the Charleston Naval Shipyard in Charleston, South Carolina. It was my first day of work as a civil engineer for a military section of the federal government, and I felt good about being able to serve my country. My father had served in the Navy in WWII and was recalled during the Korean War; there was a lot of family pride in what I was doing. At the age of twenty-two, I wanted to make him proud of me. It was also a time when the Cold War with the Soviet Union intensified as President Ronald Reagan had just become president and wanted to rebuild the military. We would nearly double the size of the Navy and would finally be providing the appropriate support equipment to make it strong.

Medical Review

On my first day of work, there were two major events in my life that took place. The first involved a physical required prior to coming on the shipyard; the other was meeting another person diagnosed with epilepsy. The first nearly crushed my career; the second led to a great friendship.

Before reporting to work, there was a medical clinic just outside the shipyard where new employees were to have a physical. This was required to determine if the person would be able to operate or even be near the equipment necessary to work on the ships and submarines being overhauled at the shipyard. The outcome nearly caused me to quit before even getting to the office where I was assigned to work.

The morning started with going through an extensive physical that was required for everyone coming to work at the shipyard. This enabled the Navy to establish a person's physical condition and validate their ability to perform the work associated with overhauling nuclear submarines and ships. It entailed hearing and vision tests, breathing tests, review of family history, addictive behaviors, and testing for exposure to lead and asbestos. These concluded with a physical with a doctor who reviewed the information from the test completed earlier in the day. Upon completing this review, the doctor discussed personal history with the employee and then did a physical involving the basics of listening to your breathing, checking blood pressure, and a hernia check.

Based on the outcome, a determination was made concerning the person's capability of performing various tasks associated with the area of work they were assigned. Essentially, they wanted to determine if a person had a physical condition that would make them a risk to themselves and others or be a liability to the government in the future. This is very important when being near or operating various machinery or being inside the components of a ship or submarine where the space can be limited and very tight.

The physical was an interesting process that took nearly a day to go through. It seemed quite a few people were hired at the same time with a particular day each month assigned to the medical staff to focus on the physicals. Doctors were brought on board to help the process for the day. There was the vision and hearing test, the process with evaluating your height and weight, and testing to make sure your lungs weren't already damaged from smoking or other form of exposure. These were the days where employers were being held responsible for damages and injuries to employees exposed to asbestos and lead.

They also reviewed the information provided by the individual seeking to work at the shipyard. The last step was filling out the documents required to obtain a security clearance to enable you to enter the shipyard. The level of security clearance depended on your area of work, and obtaining additional information and security review was completed after being hired. If you made it through all this, you were issued work boots and safety glasses and reported to your supervisor in the shipyard.

The Freak

I did really well with the physical, all the way up to the point of meeting with the doctor and completing the forms. I sat at the exam table as the doctor read through the information provided through the staff who administered the test and the questionnaire I completed concerning my medical history. Due to the arrangement of the room, the doctor's desk was mounted to the wall, and his back was turned to me. A few minutes into his review, he suddenly stood straight up and said, "Looky here, I've got me a goddamn freak." With his back turned to me, I wasn't quite sure I heard clearly what he said. I think another part of it was I couldn't believe what I heard, so I asked him to repeat himself.

This time he turned around to look me straight in the eyes and said, "You've got epilepsy, and that makes you a goddamned freak. The only thing you will be allowed to do working in this shipyard is sit behind a desk and sharpen pencils. We don't allow freaks to work here."

The doctor could not use my epilepsy to prevent me from coming to work for the federal government, but it seemed he had the power to make sure I didn't enjoy it. He was trying to discourage me from ever wanting to work at the shipyard. He completed the physical, of which I had no problem for I was in very good shape. The only exception was feeling broken inside by what he said. I could not believe I was considered to be "a goddamned freak." As I left the room, the staff provided guidance on the location of the Production Engineering Office where I was assigned to work.

Should I Quit?

As I left the building, I stopped just outside and gave serious consideration to walking to my car and driving away. I then thought it best to go meet with my assigned supervisor and tell him I would not be working at the shipyard. In the fifteen minutes it took me to walk to the office, I thought of what I would say about leaving, or should I say quitting. I was very discouraged and was thinking about heading back to my parents' house on Long Island, New York.

As I entered the supervisor's office, I didn't bother to introduce myself. I just immediately said, "I have been told by the doctor I cannot work hear, so I plan on leaving. I wish I had known this before. I would never have bothered to come." There was no way I would just sit behind a desk all day and not be allowed to oversee the work being accomplished. My supervisor had not even had the opportunity to get up from his desk to introduce himself. He surprised me by smiling and telling me, "According to me, what happened in the doctor's office has no impact on your working for me or having access to the shipyard."

It turned into one of the greatest days of my life. For instead of encouraging me to leave as the doctor implied, the supervisor explained how the doctor had no authority on my work in the shipyard. The supervisor was responsible for assigning the work and for my safety. He also told me he had another person working for him who had epilepsy. Before we talked about the work his team was responsible for, he called Mark Leyde into his office to meet me. Mark was considerably bigger than me (six feet) and very warmhearted as he smiled and shook my hand, welcoming me on board. The supervisor told Mark that the two of us had much in common, even though we had never met each other. Mark looked at me with a questioning expression, trying to figure out what he could have in common with someone he'd never met before. Then he was told, "Jon has epilepsy too." Mark smiled and shook my hand again, this time with both hands, and he did not seem to want to let go. He let me know that if I needed anything to please come and see him.

We started to share our experiences with each other, the impact of dealing with seizures, and our love of the water.

Mark

Mark invited me out to the house he rented from our supervisor on the Isle of Palms, just two blocks from the ocean and four blocks from the boat ramp to the Intracoastal Waterway. He shared the house with several interns from the University of Tennessee who worked in our section. It was a nice cinderblock house that held up well to the wear and tear of a bunch of young engineers. Our supervisor appreciated the renovations and upgrade work we did for him. Mark and I felt we could be very open with each other about our experiences dealing with seizures, the impact it had on getting through engineering school, and associating with other people. It was nice to have someone who can associate with what it is like to have a seizure and the effect it has on the mind and body. After just a few days, Mark said, "I feel like I have known you all of my life." We became best friends.

Nuclear Submarines

At work, I was allowed to do more than just sharpen pencils. My seizures were controlled with medication, and Mark helped me find the doctors necessary to get the appropriate treatment. Back at that, time treatment was simple. Just a few medications were available and not much monitoring on the blood levels. My friendship with Mark continued until his death in 2014 from a car accident; no one ever knew why his car crashed.

My supervisor gave me a tour through the dry docks where nuclear-driven fast-attack submarines were being overhauled. It was amazing to see how a submarine was brought into the dry dock—the water pumped out, and the submarine settled on a series of concrete blocks that would provide support in the appropriate place to keep it structurally sound. The blocks would also keep it from rolling over and created a tunnel to the underside of the boat where whole sections of the hull were removed to allow access to areas being overhauled.

The submarines are amazing in that they can go for months without surfacing. This is due to their power source being a nuclear reactor. While in dry dock, the reactor would be deactivated. This brought the temperatures down, yet it still required a certain level of cooling and close monitoring. There were piping systems and several backup systems in place to make sure cooling was not interrupted and to keep it safe.

I would learn about the various trades involved in performing the work and the criteria and regulations applied to make sure the systems were kept operational. Although I was fascinated with the work, it didn't seem to apply to me and my desire to move into the field of construction. Six months later, I transferred to the Southern Division, Naval Facilities Engineering Command (known as SOUTHDIV NAVFAC) Construction Division field office at the naval base.

It was a great opportunity for me as a civil engineer, for funding was being provided to upgrade and increase the size of the Navy at the height of the Cold War. My seizures were controlled with medication, and there was someone who could associate with me on what it was like living with epilepsy

Waterfront

The work with SOUTHDIV was at the field office at the Charleston Naval Base and operated by the resident engineer (civilian) and the resident officer (a Navy commander). The staff consisted of a civilian group for continuity and Navy officers for coordination with the Navy customers. I was in training and worked for another project manager and the inspection staff who taught me more about construction than I could have ever learned in a classroom. They worked with me when I had my seizure and helped me build a strong level of self-esteem.

For the first two years, I was assigned to work under a project manager who had nearly thirty years of experience overseeing construction contracts. He taught me how to maintain working relationships with the team and the importance of completing the contracts in a manner that made the contractors, customers, and the government winners. The inspectors were mostly retired construction supervisors, so they knew what to inspect to make sure the quality of the work met or exceeded the contract requirements and customer expectations. I spent many hours in the field with them learning about the techniques and quality of construction. When asked about my experience levels by customers, my response was "I just have a couple of years of field experience. However, I have a team of project managers and inspectors with over three hundred years' experience to support me."

The projects assigned to me started with the smaller renovation and upgrade to buildings that were less than $25,000. As I learned through other people's experience and demonstrated my ability to manage projects, I was given more complex contracts with higher dollar values. I was so proud to be given several projects that involved waterfront and pier renovations that would impact naval operations. To do the renovations required sections of a pier to be shut down to enable the contractors to access to the steam, water, sewer, and electrical systems being upgraded. These utilities are necessary for ships to operate and are generated by the ship while underway. Without shore power and utilities, the crew had to maintain the ship's systems. This created a fuel issue as more was needed to keep the ship ready to go to sea. More importantly, many of the crew would not be allowed to go home for they would have to stay on board to keep the systems running. Leave was very important, especially to those who had been deployed for several months to over a year. Many just wanted to go home and be with their families.

Millions of dollars of construction funding was approved by Congress for the Navy to upgrade their facilities and contracts awarded for several more projects associated with upgrading all the piers at the base. Only three had been completed, and suddenly work would be ongoing for eighteen of twenty-one remaining piers. The outages required on the utilities would simultaneously impact ship operations. Two piers were to be torn down and replaced; one new prototype pier was to be constructed. When I talked to my supervisor about this, he had me develop a presentation package to raise our concern to those who would be affected.

A meeting was scheduled with the junior officers from SOUTHDIV, the Charleston Naval Shipyard Department of Public Works, and Naval Station Ship Operations. When I completed the presentation, everyone told me this had to go up to their supervisors and commanders. Within a week, I was doing the same presentation to the supervisors and Navy commanders. They all agreed this was a serious issue, and a meeting was scheduled with the captains and the commanders involved at the shipyard and the chiefs at SOUTHDIV. We were to meet at SOUTHDIV headquarters a few miles from the naval base.

I was two and a half years out of college, delivering the message about coordinating the work with ships operations to those in the highest positions at the naval base, SOUTHDIV, and several of the captains of the destroyers and cruisers stationed at Charleston. The civilians were dressed in suits and ties and the captains in summer white uniforms. My benefit was, I had no idea who these people were or the level of their authority, so I was not nervous about presenting the issues. I was standing in front of the room and presenting a diagram of the piers with the utility outages highlighted and timelines of the work schedule. The issue was eight to ten piers would have to be shut down simultaneously to meet the schedule criteria in the contracts.

As I completed the presentation, one of the civilian division chiefs said, "Seems all the ships will have to go to sea for a while." Even I couldn't believe what I just heard, and I felt like I was going to be shot. His statement came close to this actually happening.

The room went dead quiet as the captain of one of the cruisers slowly stood up and said, "You seem to have forgotten who you are here to support. I am letting you know this building is within range of the guns on my ship." He picked up his hat and walked brusquely out of the room. The silence continued for several more minutes, and I thought the end was near. Finally, the chief of the construction division looked at me and said, "Looks like you have a lot of projects to coordinate. Make sure you do so with minimal impact to the ships."

Over the next four years, I was the assistant resident engineer or construction manager on the renovation of utilities and structural repairs to nineteen piers, replacement of two piers, and the construction of a prototype double-deck pier, Pier Zulu, which became a Navy standard. I would coordinate the schedules with the Navy Operations Division and was the primary POC for the general contractors as we worked out the schedules. Seems everyone dealing with the ship operations and public works along the waterfront would get to know me.

In our office, we had a lieutenant come on board to oversee some of the building facility contracts. He was an F-14 fighter pilot who had a vision issue that prevented him from flying fighter jets. We became friends, and he offered to take me up in a Cessna 150 to get photos of the waterfront work. The security officer gave us permission to fly over the restricted area of the naval base. The Department of Public Works (DPW) requested more photos and gave us a list of projects to photograph. When we were officially given the security clearance, we obtained two cameras and several rolls of film and headed for the plane.

We took off from the Isle of Palms and flew toward the naval base. The first project to photograph was Pier Zulu, the new prototype pier that was 70 percent complete. As we approached the naval base, I heard on the radio calls to the security office from several ships. They were very concerned with a Cessna 150 approaching the piers. There was no response from security. This went on for several minutes, and by this time, we had the nose of the plane down and were getting great photos of the construction of the pier. I was so tied up in taking the photos I wasn't paying attention to the radio calls until we heard "Request permission to open fire" from one of the ships. Then "DO

NOT FIRE! DO NOT FIRE!" "SADLER'S IN THAT PLANE!" "THAT PLANE HAS PERMISSION TO FLY OVER." At this point, we had flown so low I could see the work crew in the electrical vault on the pier and the lights on the 150-foot light poles directly across from me as the plane was pulling up. The lieutenant was totally calm about the situation and told me how he could have landed the plane with the engine stopped and the wings shot off. He assured me we would be alive; he just couldn't guarantee what we would look like. He then asked, "Should we do it again?" And I said, "Sure," as I started to change the film in the cameras.

My supervisor was terrific at keeping peace with the upper command of the agencies involved in the work. He was a motivator for me and provided guidance and suggestions at the appropriate time. Some of the most interesting parts of my role involved negotiating change orders and developing the revisions to the design necessary when unforeseen conditions were discovered during construction. I was negotiating and documenting changes of over $1.5 million as valued in 1985, supported by a well-experienced team of men who did the inspection of the work.

As the work was completed along the waterfront, a new pier was to be constructed at the Naval Weapons Station, located upriver from the naval base, for a special training facility. As part of the Cold War, the United States and the Soviet Union agreed to decrease the number of ballistic submarines capable of carrying nuclear warheads. One of these would be turned into a training facility for the officers and crew responsible for maintaining the nuclear reactors. The ballistic missile submarine was taken into the shipyard and had the midsection, where the missile tubes were located, removed. It was welded back together and made fully operational. The pier had to be completed in time to provide anchorage for the submarine and slips for the support vessels when they were ready. I was moved to the weapons station to oversee the work.

At the time, I did not know my son would be stationed there to complete his training to become qualified as an officer in charge of overseeing the nuclear reactors on the most sophisticated aircraft carriers of his time. As he told me about the facility, I kept telling him, "I know." Finally, he asked me how I knew so much, and I shared my experience. It just seemed amazing that I was allowed to be part of it, especially after what the doctor had said about my epilepsy and only ever "being allowed to sharpen pencils."

The only way this became possible was through the doctors who provided appropriate medical care and treatment and my supervisor who recognized my abilities to manage and lead. The opportunities I was provided would help me to fulfill even more positions than I ever dreamed possible.

Philadelphia Shipyard

My career with the Navy continued for another year and a half as we moved to Philadelphia, Pennsylvania, for my wife to get her graduate degree. Philadelphia had a Navy shipyard that could accommodate aircraft carriers. The Northern Division of the Naval Facilities Engineering Command (NORTHDIV) headquarters was stationed there. My wife and I lived in downtown Philadelphia, close to where she was going to graduate school. It was definitely more stressful to live in downtown Philadelphia, exemplified with my seizure and exacerbated by a long period of driving to work. There was no public transportation that could accommodate my needs. And unlike Charleston, I had to drive by myself.

I moved from working in the field and overseeing the construction of the projects to developing the design of facilities to support the families. The assignment was to become a paving specialist working on runway systems. This required going back to college and studying highway and paving design. This was a good challenge to keep my brain working hard. As my wife completed her degree, we decided Philadelphia was not for us and moved to Baltimore, Maryland. In Baltimore, there would be numerous opportunities for both our careers and proper medical care.

Chapter 6

Working for a General Construction Contractor (1989–1991)

The hell you will. If I had five of him, I'd fire the rest of you.

With my wife completing graduate school, we looked for employment in the Baltimore, Maryland, region. I had interviewed with the Navy in Washington, DC; the Army Corps of Engineers in Baltimore, Maryland; and a general contractor. The position fell through with the Navy, and the corps was very interested in hiring me; however, there was a hiring freeze. Wanting to be with my wife, I accepted the project engineer position with the contractor. The phone call from the Army Corps of Engineers came the day I was packing my belongings and leaving the Navy. The position was now available, and they wanted to talk about my start date. I thanked them and informed them they were a little late with the formal offer; I was leaving civil service to work for a general contractor in construction.

Working for a general contractor was exciting for now I would see the effort required from their perspective in lieu of the customers, as had been my experience working with the Navy. The work was more stressful, for the hours required to assemble a contract proposal and providing reports to customers often took a lot of time and impacted my sleep and eating. Stress levels increased with the worries of delivering products on time. Within a few months, our first child, Wesley, was born. And the struggle of being a father and the devotion to the employer increased my stress considerably. All these physical and emotional stressors led to my having breakthrough seizures.

At work, I was given a special assignment to develop a computer program for tracking budgets and costs on a multimillion-dollar project. Although the software existed for having a database to store all the information on such cost and budgets, the programs had to be written to produce the reports. My supervisor called me into his office and asked if such programs could be developed. Not knowing the schedule and level of importance, I assured him it could be done. Programs for construction budgets and costs were in their early stages of development, and the programs for the reports were not available as they are today.

It was a challenge that often required working many hours into the early morning. Then there was home and the child to care for. Often my fellow employees would joke about how sleep was an option we had to give up because of our responsibilities at home and work. For me, sleep was a necessity needed to control my seizures. With such stressors, the probability of my having a significant seizure increased significantly. It was only a matter of time.

Writing the programs seemed easy at first. Then the reports became more detailed, and data input had to be revised. The programs went from several to hundreds of commands. Much time was required to troubleshoot the programs and database entries for typos as either caused the reports to be worthless. I was the only person who could provide training on the data entry and the importance of not making typographical errors. The invoices were based on the direct costs of a project, so everything from buying pencils to paying staff and subcontractors had to be entered. At the peak of a project, thousands of data entries were required per month.

Seizure Breakthroughs and Job Impact

The day came when the grand mal seizure came while writing a new program to generate a detailed report. It was very stressful, for the program had to be completed and the report available within a few days. There was a very important meeting with the customer, and the company wanted to make a good impression on how they were unique in tracking budgets and costs. The aura came as I was troubleshooting the program. As much as I was hoping it would just go away, it only continued to intensify. I was safe sitting in a chair in a small room by myself, for if it was just an aura. The probability of someone noticing it happening was low.

Eventually the aura became a grand mal seizure, and many people heard me banging against my chair and table. I have no memory of my muscle suddenly tightening and my body going straight as a board as I sat in the chair. I was chewing on my tongue, and blood was dripping out of my mouth and onto my white dress shirt. My peripheral vision went away, and I could only see the computer screen in front of me. Soon it seemed to become very far away, and then it disappeared.

There was an associate standing next to me when I started to regain consciousness. She was talking to others and asking me questions. I was nonresponsive, yet I could hear and remember her telling a colleague, "Call 911." She had a look of concern on her face and kept telling other people to stay out of the room. She did not understand what had just happened and told other people medical help was on the way. My vision was turning off and on with no peripheral vision. I was not able to move or respond; however, I could hear and comprehend. I struggled with an ongoing battle occurring in my brain and had thoughts of not recovering.

By the time the paramedics arrived, my vision had returned to normal. But my speech was still impaired. They were asking me questions and trying to get a heart monitor on me. I was frustrated for I had no way to communicate. I gestured for a pen and thought, *If I cannot say anything, maybe I could write it.* This didn't work either. It was at this time the CEO came into the room. He saw me push the paramedics away and go back to the keyboard of the computer. I knew I didn't want to lose all my work and remembered to type "save."

I then picked up the phone and dialed the number to my wife's office. I clearly asked the secretary, "Is my wife there?" The secretary said, "She is out of the office. How can I help you?" The only word I could find in my mind was *shit.* After saying this, I handed the phone to a paramedic. He explained to the secretary that I had had a seizure and they needed to talk to my wife immediately.

The secretary got so excited and scared about what was happening that she had one of the other employees in her office run out the door and speed off in his car to find my wife, who was their supervisor. My wife had to calm her staff by telling them she knew of my condition and then called my office. She talked to the project manager I was working with and gave him the phone number and address of my neurologist. Since she was at the other side of Baltimore from the construction office, she asked if the company could provide transportation. She would meet us at the doctor's office.

Upon learning there was professional care lined up for my condition, the paramedics agreed not to transport me to a hospital. I was able to sign with my initials the forms necessary for this to happen. I looked like I had been in a fight, and my associate walked me out to his car. This was not a very long walk and required riding in an elevator. Even so, it felt like his car was miles away as my body hurt and was exhausted.

Due to a traffic jam, the forty-five-minute ride to the neurologist office took over two hours, and then another hour to see the doctor. By this time, I was fully cognitive and had been talking to my work associate as he drove. From the doctor's perspective, they didn't see much concerning the seizure, except the blood on my shirt and the injury to my mouth and tongue. They were more helpful with my associate and my wife's concerns as they informed them that my mouth would heal and I would be OK. They gave me a note to give my supervisor as my medical excuse. With my supervisor and the CEO witnessing the seizure, the note was not necessary.

Within a few days, I learned how the CEO had called my supervisor to his office to talk about what happened. The supervisor was nervous and feared being reprimanded for hiring a person with epilepsy. As he walked into the CEO's office, he immediately started explaining how he planned to fire me the very next day. The CEO cut him off as he said, "The hell you will. For if I had five people as dedicated to this company as that young man, I could get rid of all of you." Seems he was very impressed with my pushing the paramedics away to save my computer work, especially in the state I was in.

Job Stress

Working for a construction firm and wondering where the next dollar was coming from was very stressful, both physically and mentally. I started having more breakthrough seizures several times a week, then almost every day. My work associates knew what to do and would get up from their desk and close our office door when the seizure started. They continued with their work and talked to me when I became more cognitive. I could no longer drive, and I relied on another associate for transportation.

The computer programs I had written were working well, and the supervisor told me I would be assigned to work on a project located a few hundred miles away. My transportation would be limited, for I could not drive. I was having several seizures a week and realized I needed a more secure job that would help me with transportation limitations and would hopefully decrease the stress.

It was time to see if the Army Corps of Engineers was still interested in hiring me. I called the director of the design management branch, who remembered me from my interview nearly three years earlier. He was excited I was still interested in working for him. Within four weeks, I was officially offered the position and immediately accepted it. My job security, along with work hours, was much better than working for a construction contractor. Transportation issues were minimized, for there was a subway near my home with stops near the office. The best part was, my stress levels decreased to the point that my medication became very effective in controlling my seizures.

I had worked for the general contractor for two years and learned more about their roles in completing projects and programs. Most importantly, I was learning how stress levels played such a major role in triggering my seizures. While working for the Army Corps, there would come a time when even higher levels of stress would occur and lead to my seizures becoming intractable.

Chapter 7

The Army Corps of Engineers (1991–2015)

Your future forecast of removing the stovepipes in the agency is already happening. The person responsible is sitting beside me.
—Associate with BRAC 1995 program

My work experience as a civil engineer and project manager with the Baltimore District (North Atlantic Baltimore or NAB) of the Army Corps of Engineers (USACE) required me to be a leader. As we struggled with some of the projects we were given, I recognized the abilities and creativity of the people involved in the various phases of a project. I worked with teams consisting of a few to over one hundred people of various races, ethnicities, trades, and degrees to bring together a final product meeting the needs of the military and several other federal agencies.

As a design manager, I was responsible for the administration of multimillion-dollar contracts with design firms. Some of the projects involved great detail and planning as they were associated with medical and biological research facilities. Within two years, I volunteered to become a project manager as a new division was developed for the oversight of entire projects. This included the planning, design, and construction phases, then the turnover and follow-up with the agencies involved.

My experience with the Navy and the general contractor gave me a good comprehension of the level of effort and demands required in each phase of a project. There were many opportunities to work on projects that were very unique and demanding. For many years, I was able to control my seizures by managing my stress and taking care of myself.

The 1995 Base Realignment and Closure (BRAC)

The first major program I was involved in as a project manager involved the Base Realignment and Closure (BRAC) of Fort Ritchie. The part I was to play in was to have the facilities completed at Fort Detrick for the people to relocate from Fort Ritchie. The stress came from having to have a five-year program completed in three years. The standard manners of procurement and contract administration had to be set aside, allowing people to be more creative to achieve what seemed to be impossible. This enabled me to be creative and work closely with everyone involved. All the work for the design had to be done by our in-house staff in order to meet the schedule. Typically, the planning phase of a project was completed prior to the design starting. This enabled the requirements of the customer, any environmental issues, and the cost to be addressed and funding provided by congress to proceed. In this case, the design phase had to start prior to the planning phase being completed to meet the three-year schedule.

Often on such large programs, the design would be contracted to an architectural and engineering firm, which required five to six months to award a contract and work to start. There was no time to contract out the design of the projects, so the design was completed by the in-house design branch staff. My role as a project manager went beyond working with the other managers, for the staff had to be motivated to work overtime for six to nine months, not just a few evenings or a couple of weeks. I was amazed by how people were motivated by receiving some form of appreciation for the work being accomplished.

The various meetings I attended outside of NAB usually involved some of the higher-level management, of which I could obtain transportation. Although I would occasionally have a breakthrough seizure, the seizures were minor, and I did not lose consciousness. I made sure to keep my neurologist informed of my seizures and was prescribed new medications when needed and as they became available. My neurologist kept me on Dilantin and placed me on these as a secondary treatment.

My stress level seemed to have decreased, for the construction field staff were motivated to get the work done and beat the schedules. By working a few days a week at the construction sites and the remainder at NAB with the design team, I was able to understanding the needs of both. Meetings were scheduled and site visits arranged to obtain the information needed to keep the work moving smoothly. A couple of days a month, I was with the executive officer (XO), giving briefings to the customers and high-level management from Washington, DC.[8] The primary concern of everyone was the schedule, and I explained how the work would be completed on time.

With six months left to complete the work, I attended a meeting with the XO, who had to brief a two-star general responsible for the closure of Fort Ritchie on the status of the new work. When the general asked the XO if we would complete the construction in time for the personnel to relocate to Fort Detrick, the XO looked at me, and I shook my head yes. His response to the general was "Yes, sir." On the ride back to NAB, the XO looked at me and asked for reassurance that the work would be done in time. Knowing the people of the teams involved and their motivation to complete the program, I assured him the work would be complete on time. The schedule was met with three weeks to spare, and the move proceeded without a problem.

The Korean War Veterans Memorial (1994–1999)

As the BRAC (Base Realignment and Closure) work was completed, I was assigned as the project manager on the construction of the Korean War Veterans Memorial, on the Mall, in Washington,

---

[8]   The executive officer is the second-in-command—in this case, the second-in-command of the Baltimore District. There are five levels of those ranked as generals and are ranked from one star up to five stars depending on their level of responsibility.

DC. The design had been completed, and the construction phase was underway. The construction involved three major contracts where I was assigned as the project manager for the memorial and the contracting officer's representative (COR) on the contracts for the fabrication of the statues and the stone for the walks and mural wall. As COR, I was responsible for overseeing the work being completed and validating the progress payments to the suppliers.

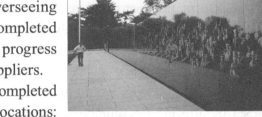

The work was completed in three different locations: the statues in Tallix, New York; the stonework in Cold Spring, Minnesota; and the memorial on the Mall in Washington, DC. I worked with some of the most renowned architects, engineers, craftsmen, and high-ranking government officials. This included presidential appointees and veterans of all parts of our military service. The most important part of this project was my love for my father, who served in the Navy during WWII and was called back when the Korean War started.

Traveling to Cold Spring, Minnesota, and to Tallix, New York, were some of the most challenging parts of the program. Traveling to Cold Spring, Minnesota, led to changes in my environment, sleep schedule, water quality, eating of fast food, and other stressors associated with travel. When I had a coworker with me, I did not worry as much about having a seizure for I did not have to drive, and there was someone who could fill in for me at the meetings if necessary. Traveling alone increased my stress level, resulting in partial seizures. On one trip to Cold Spring, Minnesota, I had several partial seizures and feared having a full complex seizure. Overall, the responsibility for managing the contracts was not nearly as stressful as the travel. I feared being pulled off the project if management found out about my epilepsy.

I believe my concerns about having a seizure enabled me to be more effective in working with various people. Often you hear about how people get nervous when they talk to someone in upper management. For me, this seemed easy compared to having a seizure. My rate of speech was excellent for doing presentations. This was actually becoming a skill set, and it was very beneficial in the next phase of the memorial. It would not be until after the presidential dedication that the most stressful phase of work would begin.

The memorial was dedicated on June 27, 1995. I did not play any role in the dedication of the memorial once the construction was complete. I did get to attend and was on the memorial grounds a few hours before the dedication by President Bill Clinton and South Korean President Kim Young Sam. I was interviewed a couple of times by a South Korean television agency, and I explained the layout and features of the memorial.

KWVM Problems

Six months after the dedication, I received a phone call from Mark, a project manager with the National Park Service (NPS). It was January 1996, and he expressed concerns about several problems they were having at the memorial. It was a few days after receiving a Commanders Award from the colonel in charge of the Baltimore District for my work on the memorial. When the colonel handed me the award, I told him I did not deserve it, for I did not consider my role to have been more than average for a project. Little did I know, the award came early for the next phase of work at the memorial required taking responsibility above and beyond anything I ever imagined.

The phone call from Mark was in reference to forty large linden trees and the piping associated with the return system on the reflecting pool. The trees surrounding the pool were dead, and the return piping on the pool was severed in several locations. Near the base of the flagpole is the dedication quote for the memorial. Some people were walking on this and slipping due to the quote being set in polished stone. Others were tripping on a small drain opening along the mural wall. There were a few cases of individuals visiting at nighttime who fell into the pool because of poor lighting. They did not get wet because the broken pipes caused the water to drain.

Soon after we talked, the memorial made the *Washington Post* and almost every other newspaper in the country. There was much criticism about the quality of the work and the Army Corps of Engineers. The next four years were extremely stressful. The architect and engineering firm hired to design the memorial developed a redesign which was rejected, for it did not address the issues in a manner that would be effective. Developing the appropriate upgrades and repairs to the memorial was now the responsibility of the engineers and contract specialist of the Baltimore District and the arborist and staff of the NPS.

Multiple Roles

I was called into the chief of engineering's office for a special meeting. He smiled as he told me I was now the project manager and the design team leader for correcting the deficiencies at the memorial. The project was now a top priority to the district commander and to himself. He let me know about having open access to his in-house design team and to inform him of any problems.

My stress level peaked the day I was assigned as the project manager and design team leader. The following Sunday afternoon, I had a minor panic attack. Within half an hour, I had an aura that continued to intensify. I was in our backyard and could not make it back to the house, so I sat down under a tree and have no recollection of what happened next. When my cognitive abilities started to return, I found myself still sitting and confused as to where I was. It would take several more minutes before I recognized the yard and the house. I was confused as the speech section of my brain was affected, and I could not find any words. As this settled and reset, some of my speech returned, and I walked back to the house. I never told anyone at home or at work what happened for fear of scaring them. This would occur two more times over the next ten days.

Within a few days, a meeting was arranged with the director of the National Park Service (NPS) of the Washington, DC region, a senior executive (SES) position or the equivalent of a general in the army. He directed his staff to provide the support needed to assure the memorial would be repaired to honor those who served in the war. The arborist with the NPS had studied the text of the original designer, rejected the redesign, and was given the responsibility for developing a design for the trees. Tracy was a pipefitter with the NPS and was told to work with me on the piping issues.

Tracy took me to every memorial in Washington, DC, that has a water system or fountain to see if there was a design that could be applied to KWVM. None of the other memorials had the same type of reflecting pool as the KWVM, so we had to develop a concept that worked and would be easy to maintain. On the back of my notebook, I drew five circles. One was large with four equally spaced inside. The large circle one represented a manhole, and the four small ones were drop baskets that fit inside to collect the debris and leaves that fell into the pool. The manholes were to be installed outside the memorial for ease of accessibility.

I went back to NAB and presented the concept to the design team. They determined the number of manholes required and the size of the piping necessary to make it work. Tracy went back to his office and had a model of the filter built to demonstrate at our meeting with the upper management necessary to obtain approval to proceed. Unlike the original design that required constant maintenance, the new design required service once a month, or worse case, once a week depending on the season. During such maintenance, the memorial would remain open and operational for the visitors.

Redesign

The KWVM had become one of the commanding officer's (CO) top three. Meetings were held regularly with the colonel and his staff. Presentations for the leadership of the American Battle Monuments Commission (ABMC), the National Park Service (NPS), and the Army Corps of Engineers were held monthly. Through the ABMC, we provided presentations to the staff of numerous congressmen, with explanations to what happened to the memorial, and the actions being taken to correct the deficiencies.

As the concepts for the renovations to the pool came together, a presentation was scheduled with the upper management of the National Park Service. It was during one of these presentations that Tracy and many other people learned about my seizures. Some sketches of the new drainage system had been developed, and a model of a collection basket was made to help explain the concept of the reflecting pool return system. I was excited and nervous—excited for the concept was relatively simple and nervous for this was a national monument. The nervousness was expounded by the fear of having a seizure—a fear I had to deal with on my own. I was sure I would lose the project and possibly my job if the upper management learned about it.

The aura started with a wave of nausea halfway through the presentation. This time it was very intense. I could feel and hear my heart racing, and my peripheral vision was gone. I knew I was going to have a seizure to an extent that would impact my ability to talk. I was overwhelmed with fear until I lost consciousness, and the room went completely black. I was later told I pounded on the table. It was an absence seizure that lasted for nearly a minute, and everyone thought I pounded on the table out of frustration.

It's amazing how the brain works. I knew what was happening with the seizure, and I knew what I had to do. I even knew what I had to say to continue with the presentation. However, I could not find the words in my brain. And if I did, I could not assemble the sentence. Within a few minutes, I could start a sentence associated with what

I wanted to state, but I could not complete it. That was when Tracy spoke up and finished the sentence for me. This went on for another ten to fifteen minutes, at which point my speech improved to where I could complete the sentence, although I was talking considerably slower. In many cases, I could not find the word for an object, so I would describe it. It was taking longer for the words to come together to express my thoughts. The upper management people were impressed with the fix we presented, and the concept was approved. It definitely took close teamwork to express what was presented during this meeting. Tracy didn't realize his role until later.

After the meeting, he came over and asked me what had happened. He was nervous and wanted to know if there was something he should do. I explained my epilepsy and that everything would be okay. He said he wished he'd known about it prior to seeing me have a seizure, for it scared him and he wasn't sure if he should have called 911. I was glad he had not. As we continued to work together through the construction of the memorial, he shared with me about a family member who was dealing with an anxiety disorder. There seemed to be similar effects between this person and myself.

In the meantime, a revised lighting scheme was proposed by a gentleman who had close relations with a Vietnam War veteran. The veteran was troubled by what was happening at the Korean War Veterans Memorial. The two of us worked closely together to develop a system that would light the statues, along with sufficient lighting on the walkways, so people could safely visit the memorial at nighttime.

As the design was completed for the renovations and the monies obtained from Congress, my role involved keeping various agencies informed of the status of the work. It was interesting and stressful wearing a suit for a meeting with high-level officials or congressional staff in Washington, DC, then go to the memorial and wear a hard hat to inspect the piping and lighting systems being installed.

Similar to the statues and the mural wall, the lighting system was not a typical construction contract, and I was made the contracting officers' representative. I was given the responsibility of overseeing the development and the installation of the system. The stress of it all, amplified by negative press releases, along with Congressional and veteran inquiries, was very high and taking its toll on me.

To bring reality back into my busy life, I received a call from my brother, who I rarely heard from. Our father had been diagnosed with stomach cancer and was not expected to live more than six months. It seemed everything came to a standstill, and the memorial was no longer my top priority. Nearly every weekend, I drove the six-hour trip from Maryland to North Carolina, where my parents lived. I thought with my seizures I would die before my parents. Now I would watch my father die. Every time I got into the car, I fought for control of my emotions. All the stress was triggering more seizures.

Fortunately, in his last few weeks, I was able to talk to my dad about life. I learned more of his service in the Navy and what he was dealing with, physically and emotionally, as his body deteriorated. He reached a stage where walking was very difficult, yet he told me he still had strength in his arms to hug me. His death came much sooner than expected—six weeks after his diagnosis. Just before his death, we were talking about his funeral service and having a flag presented for his service in the Navy. I called an associate, who obtained a flag in Washington, DC, and had it presented at the site of the future WWII Memorial and the Korean War Veterans Memorial on the Mall. They sent it on overnight mail, and it arrived the day before Dad died. He was bedridden and had no strength to move or talk. When we presented the flag, I leaned over him in his bed and gave him a hug. He struggled to get one arm over me and whispered "Thank you" in my ear as tears streamed down his face.

I had been away from the office for nearly two weeks, and the reconstruction was moving rapidly. With 70 percent of the reconstruction of the reflecting pool complete, the lighting system went from fabrication to being installed. I was asked to be the construction field engineer and manage the on-site review of both the contracts, for the inspector had been reassigned to a program overseas.

I tried to decline the offer for fear of my seizures. I was best qualified based on my knowledge of the design of the renovations and lighting systems. The only excuse was my epilepsy, and I could not tell anyone about this. This was even more difficult as I had to drive through two rush hours, as I lived north of Baltimore, Maryland.

The work required being on site at 6:00 A.M., when the construction started, and to be ahead of the snarling traffic conditions typical of the area. The lighting system was installed during the day and checked at nighttime after the sunset when it got dark. As we were in the May–June time frame, this did not happen until 9:00 PM to 9:30 PM. The testing and adjustments went on till 10:30 PM to midnight. I was tired and stressing my mental and physical being to the maximum. The date for completion had been published, and we were behind schedule for the weather was not cooperating. Management was so impressed with the lighting system for the statues and around the pool; they wanted the lighting system for the mural wall upgraded too. I negotiated the change order, and the work started immediately.

The Project from Hell

To manage the contracts and responsibilities, I found myself getting only a few hours' sleep a night. I was stressed with all the places I had to be, not to mention the level of attention the project had nationwide. At lunchtime, I would separate myself from the rest of the group, for the free time allowed me to think about something else for a moment. This helped me bring my stress level (anxiety) down. As my stress level went down, it was not unusual for me to feel an aura come, impacting my ability to speak for a few minutes. For the next several hours, finding the appropriate words associated with work took longer. I was learning to describe the object I wanted to talk about when I could not find the name in my brain.

A good rapport was developed with the NPS staff, and everyone seemed focused on getting the memorial reopened on time—everyone, but Mother Nature and the rain. Even so, the contractor's staff and all the Park Service and NAB staff worked hard to make it happen. There were no longer any disputes, only problem solving. My days were long; the paperwork and reports were completed during the weekends. The testing of the systems began as we were coming to completion. I managed to go to the beach with my family, was on the phone most of the morning, and came back to the memorial in the evenings for the light tests.

I brought Wesley, my oldest son, with me, and he was proud to be included. He even got to wear a hardhat while at the site. My sister-in-law helped by driving so I did not have to be concerned with transportation, especially late at night. It is one thing to fall asleep while driving; my concern was how fatigue is a seizure trigger.

Over the next six more weeks, the work around the reflecting pool was completed, and the memorial reopened on time. The statuary lighting was nearly complete, and the work on the mural wall lighting had just started.

It was interesting working on the lighting system and being at the Memorial at 11:00 PM or midnight. There were still busloads of people visiting the memorial. It seemed visitors from around the world were on different time schedules than we were in Washington, DC. The day came when the lighting system was completed and turned over to the NPS. A coworker was with me that day and provided transportation in a government vehicle. He saw me release my emotions as I pounded on the dashboard and cried. He never understood this was my way of releasing the anger associated with the fear of seizures. When arriving home, I was scared to relax, for releasing tension was the time I was very susceptible to an intense seizure. Seems too much stress/tension and calming down were some of my major seizure triggers.

Ten years later, I was talking to the owner of the lighting company about our experience working on the memorial. He asked me if I remembered what I said that motivated him to complete the work and make sure it was his absolute best. I was baffled as I thought about all the different things I could have said, and I was totally confounded by what the right answer might be. He went on to explain a time when we had taken a break from work and were sitting against the backside of the mural wall. He said, "You looked totally exhausted. We had been quiet for a while and trying to cool off in the hot weather when you looked right at me and said, 'This has been the project from hell.'" He thought the hell was all the work, schedules, and bad publicity. That was actually the problem; the hell was dealing with my seizures.

He went on to say he was motivated by my dedication to the project, even though it was so hard on me. If I was this dedicated to the veterans and the other people who visited the memorial, he could not let them down either. Although he was aware of my father dying a few months earlier, he was not aware that my twenty-year contract with God had reached the end. This was especially a difficult time for I had two young boys—five and seven years old—who I dearly loved. And I thought I would die soon.

A few weeks after the memorial was reopened and the lighting completed, Mark, my POC with the NPS, sent me an email with an article from the *Washington Post*. The *Washington Post* had been very critical of what happened with the memorial and the time it took to get it repaired. This article was different, as it focused on the two memorials to visit at nighttime. The two memorials referenced and reviewed were the Lincoln Memorial and the Korean War Veterans Memorial.

Loss of Friends and Coworkers

Within a few months of the completion of the renovations to the memorial, three of the key people who worked with me died. The first was Ron, who was responsible for the construction contract negotiations and contract documentation. This takes a lot of effort few people are aware of. Ron had been treated for melanoma for several years and missed one of his checkups. When he saw the doctor again, the melanoma was found in his scalp and had spread into his brain and body. He said it was stage 4 and died a few months later.

Mark was the project manager with the National Park Service. I worked closely with him to assure the work met the schedule and the needs of the National Park Service. He had a rare liver condition that developed just weeks after the memorial was reopened. He was able to come down to the memorial and see the completed systems with everything fully operational. He died a few weeks later. He was known for his kindness and work to make the Mall a beautiful place to visit. Many of the flower beds along Independence Avenue are of his design.

The third was Christine, my supervisor and mentor. We had worked together for several years, and she was providing the guidance and experience for me to move into a management position. She died of a relapse of breast cancer. Throughout this, I kept thinking I would be the one to die, not everyone else. It would be ten years before I could revisit the memorial again, for I could not control my emotions and fear of my seizures. It was after the Epilepsy Foundation Walk on the Mall in Washington, DC, in 2009.

Access Control Points and the Amputee Center

My stress level decreased significantly when the KWVM was completed, and my seizure activity decreased immensely. I would learn later that with each seizure, my brain was damaged. And my ability to control my seizures when stressed had decreased significantly.

Then came the terrorist attacks on the World Trade Center and the Pentagon, and security was being upgraded at all the army posts throughout the world. I was assigned to be the program or project manager on upgrading the security at the army posts in several states. The work involved multiple contracts associated with installing equipment thought necessary to improve security at the entrances to the post. Most of the work involved lighting, security booths, and pop-up barriers that could stop an automobile instantly.

The pop-up barriers consisted of large steel wedges where the front side would suddenly come out of the ground, creating a steel wall. Videos of the testing of the barriers showed trucks travelling at 45 mph, hitting the barriers and being stopped immediately. The result was, the cab where the driver sits was crushed as the truck was compressed by the momentum of the structure of and materials in the storage area. Cars were a little different. With a car, the front end would go under the wedge, and the occupants would be killed as the front seat went under the barrier. At this time, there were no alternative barrier systems certified for use.

After award of the contracts, new safety measures were issued requiring signals and delays to the activation of the barriers. None of this had ever been constructed, and our contracts became the test ground for all the posts within the US. As the first gates were completed, with the safety features included, it was discovered that some of these features created a safety issue too.

There were issues with equipment failure, resulting in the barriers deploying. Most were human nature, and a few automobiles were damaged. Fortunately, no one was seriously injured, for the vehicles were not travelling very fast. I was receiving calls from several facilities reporting deficiencies in the equipment. As the issues were addressed with upper management, direction was received to do extensive testing of the barriers installed at several locations. The results of the test demonstrated my concerns. I started to take the project personally, and my stress level increased significantly.

With military action underway in Iraq and Afghanistan, the number of wounded soldiers coming to Walter Reed Army Medical Center (WRAMC) had drastically increased. An Amputee Recovery Center was needed in a hurry. A cohort was assigned as the project manager, and I was assigned as the design manager. In six months, we had the design completed and were ready to advertise the contract for construction. The proposals came in above the funds available, and WRAMC was to be closed in the next Base Realignment and Closure program. Due to the need and importance of the project, Congress approved a temporary facility to be constructed.

The amputee recovery facility was to enable the wounded to be fitted for and learn to use their prosthetic arms or legs. In order to meet the tight schedule and limited funding, a new solicitation package was required within three months and the package advertised for construction. The work associated with this helped me in dealing with the stress of the barrier system contract by keeping me very busy with meeting the needs of our nation's soldiers.

It was amazing to see the wounded soldiers at WRAMC and their ability to recover. Races were held for those with prosthetic legs, and several participants were missing both legs. It was tough to see a soldier meeting with his wife and holding his baby child, with both his legs missing. Those being outfitted with a prosthetic were suffering from multiple wounds to other parts of their bodies. It was amazing to see the staff working with these soldiers and how the wounded motivated one another.

My stress level was high, and my tolerance for stress was declining rapidly. Over the next few months, the stress associated with the projects became magnified many times over by the fear of having a seizure. I was stressed out emotionally and physically, as my brain was significantly damaged by seizures. My neurologist had no other medications available for treatment; I was now having several seizures per week. During this time, I was receiving treatment at Johns Hopkins Hospital and determining if surgery was my best option.

Eventually, direction was received to stop work on the barrier system as newer and safer equipment became available. I was not present when this happened. Nor was I present when the contract for the Amputee Rehabilitation Center was awarded, because I was recovering from a lobectomy in hope to gain control of my seizures.

Section 5

Intractable Seizures and Surgery

Chapter 8

Presurgery 2005–2006

There is nothing else I can do. You need to go to Johns Hopkins.

When my seizures continued to break through my medications and treatment, my neurologist told me, "There is nothing else I can do for you, Jon. You need to go to Johns Hopkins [hospital]." Since I had been on so many medications since being previously treated at Hopkins, he told me surgery may be the most viable treatment. He gave me the contacts at one of the leading epilepsy research facilities in the world. I would become the first person with an engineering background to seek surgery as treatment of intractable seizures at Johns Hopkins Hospital. My internal medicine doctor provided the referral needed for insurance and arranged for an MRI for my first visit at Johns Hopkins. When the MRI was performed, I received a copy of it. Looking at the MRI was intriguing because there were so many images of various sections of my brain; I figured they had to indicate something.

Initial Review

I did not know who I would be meeting at Hopkins until he walked into the exam room. He recognized me right away; however, for me it took me several minutes before my brain recalled who he was. He had been in charge of the intern who provided care for me the last time I had been at Johns Hopkins. Now my stressors were considerably higher as I continuously thought about having a seizure, losing my job, or hurting my children. I wondered what his recommendation for treatment would be this time.

Everything was different. Within moments of looking at my MRI, Dr. Krauss saw the seizure trigger points in my brain. These were the lesions on my left hippocampus, which is part of the limbic system located inside the temporal lobe. After showing me the MRI, we reviewed the options available for treatment. These types of lesions or scars were typical trigger points for people who suffered from high fevers that caused seizures. The options were to continue to try to find a medication, combination of medicines, or surgery. Dr. Krauss did not think medication would be effective based on the number of years it had been applied and how the seizures became nonresponsive. Surgery was the best option.

Lobectomy

Based on the types of seizures I was having, and the lesions being identified, a lobectomy (removal of a section of the brain) seemed to be the best form of treatment. The unanswered questions were "Did the MRI show all the locations of the cause of the seizures?" and "What would happen to my ability to function when the surgery was over?" The neurologist went on to describe all the tests that would be required to verify the trigger to the seizures and validating surgery to be the best treatment.

In some ways, I was happy that we could now see the damaged area with the lesions. I was also scared about the outcome. Would I be able to learn and recall information? Would it really stop my seizures? The neurologist explained the probabilities of the effectiveness of the surgery. There was a 60 percent probability that surgery would stop the seizures. However, the numbers presented did not to take into consideration the level of education and responsibilities of the person having surgery. If I decided to have the surgery, I would be the first of my education and work experience, as an engineer, to have this form of treatment performed at John Hopkins Hospital.

Brain surgery is not to be taken lightly or to be compared to other types of surgery. The brain is the control center of the entire body, and what happens to it affects the personality of the individual. Although it may appear that brain surgery has corrected the problem, the person's personality may dramatically change. This is similar to side effects of some medications for certain people.

Survey

During my first visit, I was asked a series of questions that seemed relatively easy. The first was "Who was the previous president of the United States?" I said, "Carter." It should have been Clinton. George Bush was the current president, but I could not recall the name of Vice President Cheney. I was nervous and afraid of the outcome, which exacerbated the problems with my memory recall. More of my brain was damaged and shut down with each seizure. As I learned about the options of brain surgery, I thought about *The Silver Skates*—the Mary Mapes Dodge story with the father having reversible brain damage. Maybe brain surgery would improve my memory.

Pretest

At that time, there were four major steps to determine the extent of the surgery and the impact it would have. The first was a more detailed MRI of my brain. An MRI of the brain required the whole body to go into a narrow tube head first. I found this easier to handle if I kept my eyes shut and even fell asleep. The second was a PET scan, which is like an MRI with color that provides more information on the activity of the brain. Then a WADA test was performed to determine which side of my brain was most dominant in my daily functions, and then a week of monitoring with a continuous EEG and visuals at the hospital. The choice of proceeding with surgery depended on the outcome of the test and my willingness to have it. Overall, it would be a lesson in humility as I became more dependent on others, followed with despair and hopelessness.

Dr. Krauss then discussed what was expected of the surgery and some of the side effects. I would lose up to 10 percent of my vision in my right eye. This did not seem to make sense with the surgery involving the left side of my brain. He explained how the nerves in my eyes cross over as they travel to the optical lobe in the back of the brain; therefore the nerve attached to my right eye goes back through the left side of brain where the surgery would take place. The area affected was at the top of the eye, and he joked about my days of dove hunting and professional baseball were over. He also told the world would become a brighter place and to wear sunglasses when outside.

Dr. Krauss estimated my recovery to take six weeks for the bone and skin to heal. Up to two years of medical treatment would be required prior to considering changes to medication. In addition, it would take a considerable amount of time before I could drive. The amount of time for recovery would influence my ability to function, and work was in question. For someone who was a project manager and worked with people from various backgrounds and positions, I wondered if I would be able to comprehend all the facets of multiple projects and provide direction to the staff to keep everything on track.

Making the decision on having surgery took only a few minutes because I could not continue to live a life with seizures. The possibility of losing my job was becoming more realistic, and I nearly had a major car accident with both my children in the vehicle. I was no longer focusing on just myself; I had to consider the effect on my loved ones and friends. Seizures were dominating my life, and if I did not do something to get control, I would sink into becoming isolated and depressed. Suicidal thoughts were coming more regularly and lasting longer. I was not thinking about killing myself—I just could not find a reason to live.

Journaling

Dr. Krauss recommended that I start keeping a journal of my seizures. This helped me realize I was having two to three seizures per week. Most were absence-type seizures, where I lost consciousness for several minutes and needed to sleep afterward. I used the Navy term *pinging* when I had an aura that lasted only a few seconds. These occurred several times a day.

My memory was not the same because there were times I could not remember the names of coworkers—people I saw and talked to on a daily basis for years. When I mentioned the seizures and memory issues to a close friend, he said, "This explained why the flat look in your face is not unusual." My normal enthusiastic expression disappeared and became flat, and I looked straight forward for a moment. Panic attacks were becoming more frequent. Finding basic words was more difficult. For instance, when my wife asked me where the children were, I hesitated because I could not find the word *bed*. Eventually, I could say, "Asleep."

Mentors

To help me make a determination concerning the outcome of the surgery, Dr. Krauss provided the phone numbers of three people who had the surgery and were willing to share their experience. One was a mother busy with family, another was a truck driver, and the third was a schoolteacher. All had done well with the surgery except for the schoolteacher, who, two years later, was still on medication. We seemed to have more in common concerning stressors, and she shared a lot with me. She had a breakthrough seizure two weeks after my surgery. The wife of the truck driver offered to talk to my wife about the effects the surgery had on her husband. Everything had changed in him and their relationship as he was not the same person whom she had married. For all three, the surgery was successful, with little impact to their abilities to function. The truck driver had to be seizure-free for several more months before his license would be reinstated.

As I struggled to determine if surgery was the correct treatment, I had a dream. In the dream, I was asked, "Are you willing to help other people?" I was nervous and scared. I thought I could not help anyone because of my seizures. I responded, "I can help thirty people." I heard the voice say, "You can help 330,000." I immediately woke up and wondered, *With my seizures, how will I ever help so many people?* From that moment, I was determined to have the surgery. The answer to the question came three years later.

A Week of EEG

February came, and it was the time of seizure monitoring at the hospital. I checked in on a Tuesday morning. And after going through all the administrative paperwork, my wife and I were escorted to a room on the seventh floor. As we stepped off the elevator, I looked down the hallway and saw the main monitoring station at the entrance. As I walked into my room, I glanced around what would be my home for the next seven days. I could see a camera system in the ceiling, a bed, a chair, and a bundle of wires at one end of the room. Off to one side was a small bathroom with a toilet, sink, and shower. There was a clock above the TV, and I noted it was 11:30 AM.

From the window I could see another wing of the hospital. On top of that building was a helicopter landing pad where they brought in emergency patients. We did not immediately see or hear from anybody from the monitoring station, and my wife left at about 12:30 PM to take care of our boys. Soon after she left, a helicopter landed, and they brought someone in. I began to feel anxious and feared being locked away and left by myself. My anxiety increased, the aura started overwhelming me, and my heart raced. I was sitting in a recliner and remembered to be sure my legs were straight in front of me. I looked at the clock; it was exactly 1:00 PM. The seizure progressed for twenty minutes. I regained consciousness and stared at the clock. It was 1:20 PM. I was confused as I tried to surmise where I was. Within ten minutes, I was able to comprehend I was at a hospital but could not recall the name of it. It would take a few hours before I could remember the name of the hospital and the room being the location to be monitored for my seizures. I do not know if my speech was impeded for no one had come to orient me on the monitoring session.

At 3:30 PM, a neurologist came to talk to me about my recent history of seizures. He asked, "When was the last time you had a seizure?" I told him, "At one o'clock today." He was shocked and asked, "Why didn't you hit the call button or let someone know?" I told him I could not reasonably find or did not know what a call button looked like or what to do with it. He seemed very frustrated as I heard him say "I can't believe we missed a seizure!" several times. He immediately had a technician come in and attach the electrodes to my head; forty electrodes this time. I was wired to the wall now with a twenty-foot tether. For the next five days, I could not leave the room and was under constant surveillance and EEG monitoring. Whenever I felt a seizure come, there was a button for me to push to inform the staff. A nurse or technician would race to my room and make sure I did not hurt myself or require emergency services.

I was battling with depression as the monitoring began. For the next week, I was literally wired to the wall and monitored night and day with a series of cameras and microphones to record my seizures. I would have some privacy in the bathroom but could not take a shower. I brought several button-down shirts so I could change my clothes.

It was comforting to know the medical staff was there in case something did go wrong. My medication was reduced, and we waited for seizures to come. They hoped for a minimum of three seizures to enable the staff to determine where the seizures started and how they spread through the brain. Not every seizure would be detected for the skull protects the brain and may interfere with the equipment that measured any minor spikes in the electrical waves. I had two more auras later that afternoon that did not register on the monitor.

The next day was Wednesday, and I had two seizures and a panic attack. When I felt the aura come, I pressed the notification button so somebody would come and witness what was happening. Several times there was the aura with no detection in the system. That evening, a seizure occurred. and I lost consciousness. A staff member rushed into the room and watched me, and it was comforting to know there was someone there to care for me.

On Thursday, I hit the notification button at one thirty in the morning. I woke up briefly and said, "I am having a seizure." And I lost consciousness. The next morning, I awoke, and my mouth was extremely sore. My tongue was injured by chewing on it, along with a side of my mouth. I asked the nurse if I had a seizure in my sleep, but she had not been on staff at the time. She went back and checked the monitoring system. When she returned, she told me that I had a pretty intense seizure the night before. They were able to videotape it through the infrared camera and had the data of the EEG. The seizures were getting more intense as the medication level in my body decreased with time.

I noticed there was little difference between an aura and a panic attack. With both, there was an increased heart rate and anxiety peaks, and both affected my speech. The auras started in my stomach with a wave of nausea, and the panic attacks started with a sudden high level of anxiety.

That afternoon, the staff asked if I wanted to be part of a study that involved a mental evaluation and testing of people with epilepsy. This consisted of an IQ evaluation, memory recall, reading, and math skills. The test was not required, and there would be no charge. The purpose was to develop an understanding of how people with epilepsy adjust and function. They told me I would be the first engineer to ever consider having a surgical treatment for seizures at Johns Hopkins. I volunteered, and it was the best thing I could have done because it established a baseline to see what the impact the surgery would have to my cognitive abilities. It was more effective than I thought as the outcome of the surgery was not what was expected.

At 1:00 AM on Friday, I had a seizure that left me confused and with a headache. Later, when I woke up at 6:30 AM, I was disoriented, and a nurse came to help me figure out where I was and what was happening. Just before dinner that evening, I was talking to a friend on the phone about work and was getting stressed. I felt the aura come on and told him I had to hang up and would call him back. He asked if a nurse had come into the room, and I said, "No, I am about to have a seizure." All I remembered was hitting the notification button. When I came to about ten minutes later, there was a nurse in my room watching me and talking to me. I could not answer immediately, but the words came back thirty minutes later. It took over an hour for me to remember what hospital I was in and another three hours to remember to return the phone call. My associate was very concerned because he had not heard from me and was about to call the hospital. I told him it took this long for my memory to recall what I was supposed to do. He was relieved to know I had the seizure in a very safe place.

My wife visited me on a regular basis, and my youngest son, Steven, came once. It was difficult for the boys who, in their early teens, were struggling with their father being in the hospital and considering brain surgery. My oldest, Wes, was totally against it and feared I would never be the same or would die. Epilepsy and surgery can be traumatic for the person diagnosed with epilepsy and can have equal or even more effect on the family members. Wes had to take on the responsibility of the caregiver as he witnessed me have many seizures starting at a very young age. He did not want to come to the hospital and see me "wired" to the wall.

Saturday was the toughest day for me. I had been isolated for nearly five days and had four seizures in the past twenty-four hours. Depression was setting in as I realized the extent of my seizure disorder. A friend came to see me and was shocked by what he saw. From his perspective, he saw a close friend who loves to be outside now tied in a room with a series of wires attached to his head. He stayed for a little while and had to leave.

That night, I watched a movie about the crucifixion of Jesus Christ. The movie was gruesome, and I did not make it to the end. The anxiety set in, the room seemed to get even smaller, and there was total darkness, except for what I was seeing on the TV set. The nausea started. As it intensified, the TV screen got smaller and smaller and seemed to drift away. When I regained consciousness, I was sitting on the edge of my bed. As I regained my ability to realize where I was and what was happening, I started to cry uncontrollably. I was beaten and lost hope. This was my fourteenth seizure in just over five days—the fifth significant seizure to be fully recorded.

The Dream

I had not hit the call button this time because I could not remember to do so. Even so, someone had to come to help me. He was about my height, and unlike other staffers, he wore plainclothes and had a large wooden cross hanging from his neck. He approached me cautiously and then came closer. I wrapped my arms around his waist and rested my head against his stomach. I cried hard. I was totally overwhelmed. He said nothing and held me. Seeing the cross, the peace in his face, and his willingness to hold me brought hope back into my life. When I stopped crying and let go of him, he looked directly into my eyes and said, "It's OK. It is part of His plan." I knew then I should have total faith in God, and having surgery was only a part of my journey in life. Although I met many of the staff, I never saw this person or anyone else dressed in his manner again. In fact, he was the only person who came in and held me.

The following morning, on Sunday, the neurological medical team came in and told me I was going home that day, one day early. They had witnessed enough of my seizures to be able to make a recommendation on the treatment. My medication was increased to the normal level, and driving restrictions were imposed for several months. The technician came in and removed the wires from my head. I was elated as the freedom to move beyond the walls returned. I needed a long shower, which was required to get the adhesive from my head. It felt terrific to be clean and able to walk out the door. The ride home was boundless as I could see everything around me. Our golden retriever, Copper, frantically wagged his tail and met me as I walked in the door. I was excited to see my sons and hugged them dearly. I had a whole new appreciation of everything around me.

WADA Test

A few days later, I met with the Dr. Krauss and learned that the EEG confirmed the location of the source of the seizures. The next test would delineate the impact of having a section of the brain removed.[9] A WADA test, named after the doctor who created it, is used to determine which side of the brain is the dominant side and controls language and memory. To make this determination, each half of the brain is separately anesthetized, and the person is asked a series of questions.

The engineer in me was fascinated in the application of the test. I wondered how they would be able to apply the anesthesia to one side of the brain at a time. I discovered that a tube is inserted in the groin and fed through the arteries into one side of the brain. Once prepared, I laid down on a gurney that I would lie on throughout the procedure. A shunt was installed that would go up into my brain.

I was moved into a large room where a team of doctors and specialists prepared to evaluate my brain. First, the anesthesiologist placed the shunt into one side of my brain, and the doctors did the evaluation of my brain by asking a series of questions while one side of my brain was "asleep." The process was then repeated to the other side of the brain. As long as I kept my perspective as an engineer, evaluating and wondering how this all worked, I was not scared; in fact, I found the procedures to be fascinating.

I could see the video screen the anesthesiologist used to install the shunt as they pushed it up through the body. Although my leg had been anesthetized locally, I was amazed to see the shunt going through me yet feel nothing, for there are no nerves on the inside of our bodies that would sense this. I laughed when I realized of the fourteen people in the room, twelve were women. There I was, nearly exposed to a room full of female nurses and technicians, yet they talked about various types of makeup products. All I could see

---

[9]   Improvements in MRI imagery and neuropsychology testing have since made the WADA test rarely necessary.

of them was their eyes because of all the protective surgical clothing and masks they wore.

I was also startled by the warning signs and markers for radiological exposure. I kept looking to see if anyone was wearing a monitor—something I learned years earlier working on nuclear submarines for the Navy. It seemed there were more warning signs in the room than on the boats. When I asked the technicians, they assured me they were being appropriately monitored.

When the technicians told the neurologist I was ready, they moved my gurney to where the test was performed. The anesthesia was injected into the shunt, and I felt myself losing control. The technician from the neuropsychology section asked a series of questions that seemed easy to answer, yet what I heard myself saying sounded like my mouth was broken. I was slurring my words; they barely made sense to me, let alone the technician. After four basic questions and identifying some objects, I was moved back to the video monitor for the shunt to be relocated. It was pulled back several inches then fed through a different artery to the other side of my brain.

Once again, the same procedure was performed as before. I apparently was able to speak clearly and more precisely. And within a few minutes, the anesthesia wore off, and my memory came back. The neurologist and the technician started to walk away when I asked, "When will the test begin?" They looked at me and laughed because the test was complete. I had no recollection of being asked any questions or how I responded. From the moment the left side of my brain was asleep, there was another part of my brain in control to which I could not relate. This side performed well as my speech was uninhibited and answered appropriately—the problem being there was no short- or long-term memory.

The rest of the procedure was simple; it involved removing the shunt and stitching the area of my leg where it was inserted. For nearly an hour, I could not move to allow the blood to clot where the artery had been cut.

As I was travelling home, a flood of thoughts overwhelmed me. I was intrigued by the techniques that were applied for the test and the number of people required for the procedure. The equipment and the skills of the people involved were beyond what I ever thought possible. I was fearful of the outcome and the recommendations the neurologist would provide. I wondered, *If they took out my left hippocampus, would the person I know be gone?* Some of the answers would come the following week when I had my appointment to see the Dr. Krauss to learn the outcome of test and the impact brain surgery would have on my personality and abilities.

When I met with Dr. Krauss, he was excited. He explained I did well with word memory, math, and reasoning when the left side of my brain was anaesthetized. The difficulty was not having any memory of the event. When the right side was anaesthetized, my ability to do math was affected as I mixed the sequence of the numbers. I could not find the words for a *protractor* or a *peacock*, and my speech was slurred. To have a section of my left hippocampus removed made sense, and I told him I would like to proceed with the surgery.

Self-Treatment

The surgery was scheduled for May 15. At work, I talked to my supervisor, who was aware of my seizures and some of the problems I was having, especially with transportation and some difficult days performing at work.

My ability to remember what I was working on was becoming more difficult. When the topic changed, I struggled to understand what was being discussed, if I was able to at all. I had drastically increased my dosage of medication to get the seizures under control, and I could only imagine what the higher dosage was doing to my liver and kidneys. It also changed my personality because the old Jon, who rarely got angry, would verbally explode over seemingly insignificant things.

All I had to do was survive for the next five weeks till surgery. I was thoroughly convinced surgery was my only option for treatment. Would I be in the sixty percentile with my seizures stopped or in the forty percentile requiring medication? My hopes were totally focused on the surgery and prayer.

The Amputee(s)

Five days before surgery, I had a meeting with Rick about completing the documentation for the award of the Amputee Rehabilitation Center at Walter Reed Army Medical Center. Rick worked in the construction division and struggled with cancer in his leg for many years. His leg was now three times the size of his other leg. Similar to my situation, there seemed to be only one answer: proceed with surgery.

He was sitting in his cubicle, staring at his leg and struggling with his emotions. He felt broken. He didn't even recognize me standing in his doorway, so I asked him what was happening. He continued to stare at his leg and fought back tears as he told me about having to have his leg amputated. My response was "That's easy. I'm having a section of my brain removed on Monday." His head jerked up as he quickly looked at me with an expression of disbelief. That's when I told him I was having brain surgery to get control of my seizures. We stared at each other in silence and then began to laugh together.

The longer we laughed, the harder we laughed. Neither of us had laughed that hard in years. We laughed till we cried. We laughed at ourselves and our situations. Each of us had felt sorry for ourselves and now discovered someone who had it just as rough. He was smiling as he got out of his chair and walked over to shake my hand. As he approached me, we did not put out our hands; we embraced each other for a long hug. We laughed once more and wished each other the best with what our futures held for us. Upon returning to my office, I realized we never addressed the questions about the contract award for the amputee center.

Family Support

Over the weekend, my wife and I tried to celebrate our twenty-fourth wedding anniversary. It was hard because surgery was scheduled for Monday morning. On Sunday afternoon, the pastor of my church came to pray with me and learned more about what was to happen the following day. I had no idea if I would be the same person as before or if a part of me would die. Yet I had faith everything would work out. Prayer was a powerful tool that got me through the situation.

I wrote a letter to my sons in my notebook for them to find if anything went wrong. I wrote this:

> There will be anger and frustration in life, but do not let these become you. Use them as guides and never give up hope. You are gifted and can do whatever you like with your life. Stay focused and use life challenges as a guide to build a good and strong character. Never let disappointment get you down for long.
>
> Love Dad

Chapter 9

Surgery

As long as I have an ounce of hope, I can get through anything.

It was the Sunday night before surgery, and the hospital was very quiet, especially in the neurology test center where the MRI was to be performed. Tags were placed on my head. Once more, my body went into the isolated narrow tube of the MRI. When I went home, I had tags on my head to help the surgeons follow the map the MRI created of my brain.

The morning of surgery was relatively simple. All I had to do was check in and report to the surgery center. This seemed odd in some ways. Previously, each time I had been in the hospital for the presurgery testing and doctor visits, I was very nervous about the outcome. This time, there were no other options if I wanted to continue to live a full life.

The surgery was delayed four hours due to an emergency procedure the surgeon was performing. Late in the morning, I was taken to a room to change my clothes into surgical attire. Another pastor of my church came to see me in the presurgery prep room, and my wife was able to follow her in. She prayed with me. I struggled with my emotions as I said goodbye to my wife as I was taken into the preparation room.

In the preparation room, the anesthesiologist talked about the process of applying the anesthesia and had me sign some documentation. My fear of losing *me* had not been abated. I had no idea who I would be after surgery. Having a section of my brain removed could impact my abilities to remember and recall, or it could change my personality altogether. Would my soul still be with me as I was transformed? As the anesthesiologist put a mask on my face and started to give me a general anesthesia, I followed his instructions and started to count backward from one hundred. I made it to ninety-eight. This was all I remembered for the next twenty-four hours, even though I was awake for several hours that evening and throughout the night.

Surgery

A section of my hair was removed for the surgical incision. The embrasure started just behind my left ear, going up slightly toward the back of my head and following the curvature of my skull to half an inch from the hairline along my face. The incision cut a bundle of nerves that controlled the sense of touch along the left side of my face.[10]

A two-by-three-inch section of my skull was sawed open, and a section of my left temporal lobe was removed to provide access to the hippocampus. This is narrow and runs toward the middle of the brain. The doctors were able to track and remove over two-thirds of it, leaving an open tunnel where it once was. The autopsy revealed how it had hardened and was minimally to no longer functional. The hardening was the outcome of the many seizures that took place and, in engineering terms, welded it all together.

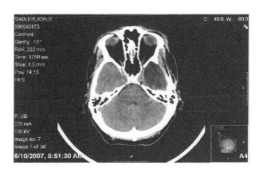

Postsurgery

On Tuesday, the day after surgery, I was monitored in an ICU. I could not figure out where I was or why I had some object attached to my face. I kept pulling it off, and some lady who was near me

---

[10] It was amazing how the nerves grew-back together over the next several months. Now when I touch my chin, I feel it at the top of my head.

would say something and put it back on. At the time, I had no idea she was a nurse who specialized in the ICU, nor could I comprehend what the breathing mask was on my face. She must have been getting frustrated with me, for soon after she would return to the monitoring station, I would take the mask off again. This process happened time and time again.

I later learned an MRI was done soon after surgery to make sure there was no internal bleeding. There was none; however, an air bubble was discovered. Oxygen was used to make the air bubble go away. Now I know what they mean by a "bubblehead."

Later that afternoon, I was moved to a regular room for a couple of days of monitoring and recovery. The recovery team told me to push a button along the inside of the bed if the pain became too unbearable. Yet due to my surgery, I had no memory of being told this. A few hours later, the pain was starting to become uncomfortable, and I could not remember to push the button or even how to call the nurse. The pain was not from the work on the brain; it was from the area of the skull and skin that had been cut opened. I just had no short-term memory and could not recall what to do when the pain became intolerable.

Several neurologists came into my room to check on me. They asked me the same basic questions.

"What is your name?"

"How old are you?"

"What day of the week is this?"

"What is your wife's name?"

"Where are you now?"

"What is the name of the hospital?"

Fortunately, I could recall my name, and especially my wife's name. It would take another day for me to remember the day of the week and the facility I was in being a hospital. I could not remember the name of the hospital. They would tell me, "This is Johns Hopkins Hospital." The question was repeated a few minutes later, and I still could not recall "Johns Hopkins." Eventually I learned to recall part of the name by associating it with my own—Jon and Johns. It would take several more weeks to recall the whole name. The neurologist who worked with me in my week of EEG monitoring came several times and seemed disappointed.

Impact to the Senses

Later that day, I was given a salad and hamburger for lunch. It was the first food I had in over forty hours. Even though my stomach was empty, I was not interested in any food. The hospital staff thought it essential and wanted me to eat. I bit into the hamburger and could only taste salt. I could not believe they would give me such salty food. As it turns out, my sense of taste was temporarily impacted by the surgery and swelling of my brain; salt was the only flavor that registered in my mind. Since it was the only flavor I could taste, it was intensified a hundred times over. The salad seemed buried in salt too. And in my frustration, I threw part of it off the tray. I would have tossed it farther if I could have remembered how to throw. Dinner was lasagna that felt like it burned my mouth and throat. It was not from the heat; it was how my brain registered the taste. The words necessary to explain my situation were not there in my head, and I could not verbally respond to my wife or nurse about why I was angry.

Dr. Krauss came to see me soon after being relocated from the ICU. After asking me how I was feeling, he asked, "What's one hundred minus seven?" In my mind, I could not figure out what he meant by one hundred or seven, let alone minus. After a few minutes, the number ninety-five popped into my mind. I was not sure what it was; however, it seemed to register with the question the doctor asked, so I said, "Ninety-five." Suddenly, I felt that it was incorrect and said, "No, that's not right." Another minute went by, and the number ninety-three popped into my mind. I said, "It is ninety-three." The doctor then asked, "What is ninety-three minus seven?" Again, I was baffled, then suddenly the number eight then eighty-eight came to my mind, and I said "Eighty-eight." There was this sensation that eighty-eight was not correct, and I corrected myself by saying, "No, that's not right." The number eighty-six suddenly appeared and seemed correct, even though my immediate thought was, *What is eighty-six?* I then said, "Eighty-six." The doctor asked, "What is eighty-six minus seven?" My mind suddenly recalled all the numbers starting with eight, from eighty to eighty-nine. Taking seven away from eighty-six was less than eighty, but what was the number before eighty? After what seemed like forever, the seventies came, and I answered, "Seventy-nine." The doctor said, "Minus seven." My brain was stressed, and I was getting tired. The number seventy-two came quickly. "Minus seven," and I could not recall the sequence of numbers that came before the seventies for several minutes. Then the number sixty-five came to me, and I answered. The moment I answered, I heard, "Minus seven." The number sixty was not enough, and suddenly the number fifty-eight registered, and I answered, "Fifty-eight." "Minus seven." I immediately said, "Fifty-one." "Minus seven." By this time, my head severely ached, and I was exhausted. When I finally found "forty-four," the doctor said it was time to take a break, and I fell right to sleep.

Cognitive Testing

My inability to remember how to apply the pain medication became a concern, and the psychology department was called to perform a test of my cognitive skills and memory. The test was relatively simple and consisted of pictures of items someone of my background should easily identify. The ones I could not answer were a protractor, a compass, and a trellis—essentially anything associated with engineering. I recognized them; I just could not find the name of the objects, indicating significant memory issues. When it came to names, I did well with family members; however, I could not remember the name of my neurologist or surgeon or the name of the hospital I was in. I felt dumb, and the pain in my head was now intense. The technician could not allow me any pain medication until the test was complete, for it would impact my cognitive skills.

The technician told my wife I would need extensive therapy that would start in a couple of weeks. I disagreed, my problem being I could not find the words to express myself, but I knew they were in my memory somewhere. The nurse came in and once more explained to me how to apply my own pain medication. For the next twelve hours, the nurses provided the pain medication. After that, Tylenol was given at mealtime and worked well. Later that afternoon, my sister-in-law brought me a chocolate milkshake, and it tasted great. Later that evening, I asked the staff for ice cream. They gave me both vanilla and chocolate, and they tasted wonderful.

Late that evening, the surgeon came into my room and removed the catheter. He then told me to slowly sit up and helped me get out of bed. As I stood beside the bed, my balance seemed off, and I was afraid of falling. We talked about this, and after a few minutes, he said, "Let's go for a walk." I had some difficulty getting started, and he held my arm. It was exciting to be able to move. I walked slowly as we did a lap around the nurse's station. Around that time, my wife came, and I asked the doctor if I could do another lap. He was glad I wanted to, and my wife helped me. It felt good to move even though my head hurt so much.

The next day started as a team of doctors came into my room and did another examination. Once again, I could not provide any names of the doctors or of the hospital I was in. Later, the surgeon came in and asked me what his name was. I could not tell him, so he took his glasses off and asked me to identify the parts. Instead of saying *bridge*, I said *nosepiece*. I could not come up with the name for the hinges or frame. The lenses I identified as glass. He was using the parts of the glasses as a way for me to remember his name. The process he introduced me to would not take hold until several weeks later.

I was kept an extra day due to concerns with some of my blood test. This I associated with not eating for several days. The food improved as my sense of taste came back. I could taste more than salt, and I remembered what good food really tasted like. I was looking forward to getting out of the hospital and disappointed I could not leave.

When Thursday came, I got to go home. I was so happy, and my headaches were now at a tolerable level. I could smile again and feel good. Before leaving, a manager on the hospital nutrition staff came to see me to get my opinion about their service. I wanted to talk about how my surgery impacted my sense of taste. The old Jon wanted to put everything into a brief synopsis of each meal, the quality of the food, and when it was delivered. I struggled for a while, trying to put the sentences together. Some of the words appeared; however, they would not come together. The idea was there; I just could not say it. I finally looked at the technician and said, "It sucks."

She was so surprised by my response being so blunt she did not know how to respond. She eventually apologized and asked if I could share some of the details. My wife explained my surgery and the difficulty I was having putting sentences together.

A few hours later, I was discharged from the hospital. As I rode home in the car, I was amazed at what I was seeing. I had a new perspective of all the buildings and people we passed and the colors in the sky. It was like I was seeing it for the first time and was so appreciative of what I could see. I was excited to know my older sister, Susan, who lived in North Carolina, was waiting for me at home. She would be shocked when we first saw each other.

When I walked into the house, she saw me and asked how I was doing. In less than a minute, I told her everything I had been through over the past few days. We were both shocked. She stood staring at me, and her mouth fell open as she had difficulty registering what was being said to her. I was surprised for I was speaking in complete sentences at a rate of speech twenty times faster than ever before. The words came to me without any thought. Everything made sense if you could conceive everything I said at such a rapid pace. Imagine taking a recording and speeding the playback way up, similar to what you hear at the end of an advertisement on the radio where they speed up what they have to say to be within the time allotted. That was how I was speaking. I had only a brief memory of what was said.

When the boys returned from school, I was beaming with joy. I recognized them and knew their names. I could remember everything about them. They were so happy I was home and looked so good. They were with me physically and mentally. I had returned.

Chapter 10

Recovery (2006–2009)

Though my body appears whole, the operation and control center of my brain is damaged. It can only be fixed by the demand to rewire . . . work with me.

The section of my brain that was removed included the forward section of the left temporal lobe that provided access to the limbic system where the hippocampus is located. The surgeon removed two-thirds to three-fourths of the left hippocampus. In simple terms, the hippocampus is the data control center or, in computer terms, the RAM of the brain. The left side of the brain processes or dominates the technical or analytical information we are exposed to. This is the part that processes the information obtained through reading, listening, hearing, etc. and stores it away in the frontal cortex or database of the brain.

When the information is needed, the hippocampus recovers it and processes it accordingly to the situation at hand. To explain this to my friends, I had them imagine a library consisting of hundreds of floors with staircases to access thousands of files at each level. From the first floor, one can see the various walkways that go around each level with ladders extending from one floor to the next that appear to go on for infinity. There are walkways and railings on each floor with rows of files lining the walls and extend deep into each level in neat rows.

The surgery in my brain left many ladders torn from the wall and damaged file cases and torn files laying everywhere. As you look further, you see more levels of damaged ladders, some impossible to climb. Others will take a lot of effort and time to climb. Most of the files still exist, only there is no longer any access to get to them.

It seems difficult, if not impossible, to get to any of the appropriate levels to store or retrieve information.

A week after surgery, I could read a sentence; however, the words made no sense. I could not remember anyone's name outside of a close friend and family. Five days after surgery, Susan was reading the comics in front of me, and I could see the Word Scramble problems upside down on the back of the paper. When she was done reading the comics, she asked me how I was doing. In response, I answered all four of the word scramble problems. She was shocked again, for this was the first time I had done the word scramble.

The left side of my head still hurt, and I could not straighten my right leg. My stretching exercises I did for running prior to surgery were nearly impossible to perform. I wondered if I had a seizure during the surgery, for this was when my body was restricted from moving. My memory was a mess. And during the second week, I could only recall the names of two of the twelve people I worked closely with from my office. The others would take over five weeks to return. In three weeks, I found Sudoku in the newspaper and started doing the puzzles. I could do the first level in a couple of hours. On Tuesday, the next level was issued. This would take several attempts and many corrections. I gave up on Wednesday through Friday for they were too difficult. My head hurt as I would not give up and pushed myself for hours. It would be several months before I could do the most difficult level, even then (and now this takes time). Exercising my brain was similar to doing a heavy physical workout. Within a few hours, I was exhausted and was sleeping ten to twelve hours a day and taking naps.

During the fourth week, a friend from church had me go with him as he travelled in his work around the county. I was intrigued by what I saw and the people I met. In many cases, I could not find all the words to complete sentences as I shared my experience with other people. Other times the words came out of my mouth very quickly, and then I struggled to remember what I said.

Word Recall

School had ended for Wesley and Steve, and we went to the beach for a week. I felt great walking on the beach, even though I could not do what I typically would, such as swimming and sailing. I started to regain weight as my sense of taste returned and my appetite improved. I was now eating vegetables that I did not like prior to surgery. My head no longer hurt, and I was more attracted to my wife.

Prior to surgery, I was predominantly right-handed. Without thinking about it, I picked up my fly rod with my left hand and started doing a practice cast in the backyard. It took some time before I realized I was using my left arm and reaching my target with little effort. I switched over to my right hand and did equally as well. Curious as to what was happening, I ran into the house, picked up a pen with my left hand, and started writing. I was amazed how it required little concentration and felt natural. The difference between using my right or left hand was how tired my left hand became after a short period of time.

Brain Exercise

Things were going so slow in my recovery that it seemed impossible to be able to do what I had done prior to surgery. I was sleeping over ten hours a day and taking naps when I did something that made my brain have to work, like reading. The engineer in me started to attempt to understand what was happening as I decided not to give up, and I started searching for a means to access my memory.

Just prior to surgery, I had learned to play "Amazing Grace," written by John Newton in the 1800s on the piano. Now, as a challenge to myself, I started working on memorizing the words. The words hit home in many ways to me, just not through the same kind of life events. It would take four weeks of repetitive writing, reading, and singing to remember the first stanza:

Amazing Grace how sweet the sound
That saved a wretch like me
I once was lost, and now am found
Was blind, but now I see

The words I struggled to remember were descriptive or nouns. I could always recall "Amazing Grace." The words I struggled with were *sound, wretch, lost,* and *found.* The tune I had no problem remembering.

The more I worked at memorizing words, the more I could remember. It was like building a new ladder to get to the appropriate floor of the library in my brain. Building the ladder took time and a demand to do so. The effort included sorting through the damaged files in my brain and opening the ones that were still whole. New paths would develop to access the information. This required a lot of effort, and the paths closed off as I grew tired. The more tired I became (and become now), the more difficult to recall the words, even though I may appear to be doing well physically. Tiredness and sleep improved with time. The doctors said recovery would take up to two years. For me it would be closer to ten years.

Fear Impulses

As I was rediscovering how my brain worked, I started to have panic attacks and be overwhelmed with fear when venturing outside the house. Flashbacks of being in the hospital or immobilized in an MRI unit were common. The fear of not being able to breathe came daily as I my nose became stuffed from hay fever. I just could not remember to breathe through my mouth. It seemed everything was amplifying the fear center (amygdala) of my brain. I would taste foods when I was not eating, smell things that were not near me, and feel like there was a hole in the back of my sinuses as I breathed. The side of my head began to feel strange. I would later learn these were all forms of seizures.

Nerve Reconstruction

There was a bundle of nerves that was affected by the surgery where the scalp and skull were cut to access my brain. As my head healed, the nerves began to come together, and the sense of touch was returning to an area around my mouth and chin. However, they were not reconnecting in the right order, because when I touched my chin, I felt it at the top my head. When I flossed my front teeth, I could feel a tingling pain near the top of my head.

As I discovered ways to get my memory back, I pushed myself harder. Although my body was not tired from the brain exercises, my brain was. The auras came back, and I was very scared of having a full seizure as my heart rate would go up. I would stop what I was doing and walk away from where I was working (to change the environment), and the aura would stop. Going back to work led to an aura nearly every time I took on a project I had previously been working on. This happened many times while talking with cohorts at work; however, I noticed my speech was not affected as in the past. It would take several years of exposure to the past and people to stop the auras. The setback was, I was having more auras after surgery than before, just not losing consciousness.

One evening, a neighbor asked me how I was doing. We started to talk about what had happened with seizures and surgery, and she kept wanting to know more and asking detailed questions. As I shared more of the details, I was hit hard with an aura that raised my anxiety level, and my heart raced. I told her we had to change the subject for I was not feeling well. She started to ask me what was happening, and I walked away to change the environment. I was conscious the whole time, and within a few minutes, the aura stopped.

Loneliness

I needed someone to talk to about what was happening—someone who could relate to what I had been through and what was happening now. I could not tell my family about the auras for it may seem the surgery was a failure, and they did not want me to have it done in the first place. There was no one I knew who could relate to what epilepsy was like. I would walk with my golden retriever to the woods nearby where I could hide and cry out loud. I kept praying and asking God, "What am I supposed to do with this?" I thought I had been in the darkest time of my life prior to surgery, and now it was getting even darker. There had to be a meaning and a purpose to my experience.

I was learning about myself as I started to memorize the second stanza to "Amazing Grace." It did not take quite as long as the first— only about two weeks to memorize. The words in this stanza applied to my current situation. I was buried in the fear of the outcome of the seizures and surgery. All I needed to do was to believe, and my fears would be relieved.

> 'Twas Grace that caused my heart to fear
> And Grace my fears relieved
> How precious did that Grace appear
> The hour I first believed

I had a difficult time when I sang the first and second stanzas together. It seemed it would take three to four attempts to be able to sing through both without missing a word or hitting a dead end in my brain. The phrase *dead end* seemed to make sense, for it seemed my memory would go down the old path and hit the end created by the surgery. When this happened, I had no idea how the song continued. I learned how frustration magnified the problem.

Control took exposure to the things that were triggering my mind to go into the panic mode. I returned to my workplace at the Corps of Engineers to let people know I was still alive and would be out for a while. When I walked into the chief of engineering's office and approached the secretary, I had a seizure. It was just four weeks after surgery. My aura started, and I could not find the words I wanted to say. She started by saying it was nice to see me again and how she was the only person in the office at the time. This was a good thing, for it took a few minutes before I could assemble the sentence I wanted to say. This was my first simple focal seizure after surgery.

I returned home as quickly as possible and sat on the couch in disbelief of what happened. In some ways, it was good, for the secretary could now let everyone know it may be a while before I was able to work at the office. I was discouraged, for I knew I was not in the sixty percentile of being cured.

That afternoon, a friend was taking me out to the Scout camp where my youngest son, Steven, had been camping for a week. It could not have come at a better time to be with my son in a setting away from home. My fears were quieted as my mind became busy with something important, and I was in a safe area with a friend and my son. It was time to memorize the third stanza of "Amazing Grace."

> Through many dangers, toils, and snares
> I have already come
> 'Tis Grace that saw me safe thus far
> And Grace will see me home

Frustration no longer dominated as the words came together. When I could remember any of the three stanzas, I smiled. When I remembered all three together, I smiled and cheered quietly. I was smiling a lot more often.

Psychological Testing

Through the recommendations provided by the speech therapist soon after my surgery, I returned to Johns Hopkins Hospital Neuropsychology Department. It had been three months since the surgery. I met with the neuropsychologist for a discussion prior to the testing being performed. He was impressed with my recovery and looked forward to seeing the results of the test.

The parts of the test that seemed extremely difficult involved remembering names and identifying objects. I had scored low prior to surgery in the thirty percentile. This time I scored the lowest possible—in the less than one percentile. Verbal memory and what was being told to me had declined. Prior to surgery, I could glance at a code of eight digits, consisting of numbers and letters, and type it into a computer. Now I had difficulty remembering two digit numbers and was reversing what I was hearing. Identifying objects was difficult, and I still could not recall the names of a "compass," "protractor," or "trellis."

The fascinating part was my ability to problem solve had improved. This was through the use of figural learning, where my cognitive skills of hands-on application had immensely improved. For instance, the correct answer was not always chosen; however, on the side of the question, I had written out the correct manner to solve it. My ability to problem solve had improved slightly. This was very important in my recovery. Memorization and reading were poor to begin with; now those skills were even worse.

The most amazing part of the test was how my brain was working faster than before surgery. The damaged section removed, it was processing information significantly faster. No wonder I could talk faster now. At the end of the test and the interview, it was determined my own manners of treatment were enabling my brain to heal and have good control of my cognitive abilities. It would just take time, maintaining a positive attitude and a demand for my brain to map new ways to find/recall information.

Neuropsychological Performance
Surgery May 2006

	Preoperative February 2006	Postoperative July 2006
General Intelligence (IQ)	87th	88th
Language		
Naming	31st	<1st
Fluency: Initial Letter	10th	9th
Fluency: Category	32nd	9th
Verbal Memory		
Total Learning	16th	5th
Delayed Recall	4th	14th
Recognition	55th	10th
Figural Learning		
Total Learning	62nd	90th
Delayed Recall	82nd	>93rd
Recognition	>16th	>16th
Processing Speed	58th	70th

Interview

A few weeks later, I was asked if I would be willing to share with the hospital staff the outcome of my surgery and what it was like dealing with seizures. Every week, the staff of the neurological department would have a conference meeting during lunch and would appreciate my being interviewed. I immediately agreed, even though I was still suffering with agoraphobia. The only way to recover from this was through exposure. When I arrived at the chief of neuropsychology's office, we talked for a few minutes and proceeded down to the conference room. The stage was the lowest point, with the seating rising on a very steep incline. This allowed everyone to easily see the people being interviewed. Another advantage was those on the platform could easily concentrate on one another and the subject matter, for you could only see the first couple of rows of people without tilting your head back to see above yourself.

I was told how the meeting would go and was set up with a wireless microphone. The assistant chief of the neurological department would do the interview as the chief was not available this time. The assistant chief and myself were to sit on the side of the first row until introduced. Then we were to walk to the center of the stage, where there were two seats facing each other. All I had to do was pay attention, follow the lead, and answer the questions to the best of my ability. If I became too nervous, I was to let them know, and they would not require me to participate.

The hall began to fill up as it got closer to the start time. I recognized the lead neurologist and neurosurgeon who worked on my case. I also recognized some of the nursing staff and those who served the food. The lighting was dimmed as the session started. The only section with lighting was the stage. Then a picture of my brain, over six foot by six foot, appeared on an overhead screen. I was mesmerized by it as the Chief of Neuropsychology talked of several other items of the week and then proceeded to talk about my case history. We were introduced and proceeded out to the chairs.

I was extremely nervous, and my hands started to tremble. While looking at the picture of my brain, I started to have auras that lasted ten to thirty seconds, and I feared they would progress into a full seizure. All I thought about was "How can I get through the interview without having a seizure?" Once seated on the stage, the interviewer demonstrated a manner of kindness and appreciation that helped calm me down. As I talked of my experience, the amygdala, or fear center, in my brain began to calm down. I started to remember the presentations I had done to congressional staff about the Korean War Veterans Memorial and all the meetings I chaired involving numerous engineering staff, customers, and upper military staff. The old Jon was discovered and started to look up into the audience and find the staff involved in the various stages of my treatment. I was enjoying talking directly to them. As we came to a close, I was asked what I would recommend to the staff. My conclusion was not to feed someone a hamburger so soon after surgery and be aware of the impact surgery may have on a person's short-term memory.

When time came to leave the building, I felt much better and began to believe I was on my way to recovery. I would learn how rewiring the brain takes time. Like learning a line to a song, it requires multiple attempts and repetitions. Although my fears were calmed as I was in front of the group, the fears quickly returned and seemed magnified as I left the building. It would take several years of exposure and academic study to regain my confidence and be a leader again.

Church Support

The leadership in the Reisterstown United Methodist Church, where I had been a member for several years, assisted in my recovery. I was asked to join one of the pastors in a meeting with several other people. She started the meeting reading Matthew 17. Matthew 17 is about Jesus being transfigured on the mountain, where two of his disciples are with him when they witness Jesus with Moses and Elijah. They see his face shine like the sun and his clothes become pure white. They hear the voice of God, and Jesus tells them not to be afraid. The reading continues as Jesus comes off the mountain and sees his other disciples and a crowd of people:

> [14] And when they had come to the multitude, a man came to Him, kneeling down to Him and saying, [15] "Lord, have mercy on my son, for he is an epileptic[c] and suffers severely; for he often falls into the fire and often into the water. [16] So I brought him to Your disciples, but they could not cure him."

¹⁷ Then Jesus answered and said, "O faithless and perverse generation, how long shall I be with you? How long shall I bear with you? Bring him here to Me." ¹⁸ And Jesus rebuked the demon, and it came out of him; and the child was cured from that very hour.

¹⁹ Then the disciples came to Jesus privately and said, "Why could we not cast it out?"

²⁰ So Jesus said to them, "Because of your unbelief;[d] for assuredly, I say to you, if you have faith as a mustard seed, you will say to this mountain, 'Move from here to there,' and it will move; and nothing will be impossible for you. ²¹ However, this kind does not go out except by prayer and fasting."[e] (New King James Version)

The pastor was using the reading to talk about how we can change if we believe. The moment she finished, she looked at me, and her face started to flush as her mouth dropped open. She immediately realized the reading included how difficult it was to cure a child with epilepsy and started to apologize to me. The seizures were considered demons because they were so difficult to understand, and often the cause is unknown. She was afraid I took my seizures as a form of possession. I assured her everything was fine with what she read. I had never heard this passage from the Bible before and was amazed.

Here was a child with intractable seizures, living in a society that did not understand epilepsy. The explanation of a seizure was possession by an evil spirit. Treatment came through rejection and isolation of the person thought necessary to keep other people from having seizures too. The boy suffered more from society's view of his condition to the extent he attempted suicide many times. The demonic possession was not of the boy but of the people who feared him, the demon being fear. There are similarities to this story in today's society—the difference being we understand seizures are not caused by demonic possession. They are due to an injury, structure, or chemistry of the brain. Isolation still exists for the same reason because most people do not understand seizures.

I started to think about what the boy did when he no longer had seizures and had many questions. His father witnessed what happened in the child being healed, but did the child still fear having a seizure? Could the child learn and remember new things? Did he use his life as a representation to others that they can keep moving forward too? How would others who witnessed his seizures accept him? The time would come when the answer would be provided as events and interactions with other people began to happen.

I started memorizing the fourth stanza of "Amazing Grace" with the focus on hope and endurance:

> The Lord has promised good to me,
> His word my hope secures;
> His will my shield and portion be
> As long as life endures.

Memorizing the fourth stanza took only a few days. I was smiling more and laughing when I could sing all four stanzas. I realized I still had an ability to remember words and learn by not giving up. The fifth stanza came even easier.

The church had a men's group I had helped establish through the direction of the pastor. The men prayed, visited, and challenged me. One of the fellows also led the contemporary service and asked if I would lead the prayer session at the next service. There was a time when we would have the congregation share their joys and concerns and then pray together. The leader would make a record of what people shared and include it in a prayer. The prayer closed with everyone saying the Lord's Prayer together. I quickly agreed to do this for I needed the exposure to get over my fears.

Over the next couple of years, I would do the prayer once per month. It would take me several hours to write a prayer that was just a few minutes long. The prayer started with asking the congregation to share their joys and concerns. I was challenged in addressing everyone's joys and concerns as people raised their hands and expressed their concerns or what they were thankful for. I tried to jot down the key points, like the name of the person or place I needed to include in the prayer. While leading the prayer, my whole body shook with nervousness. Most people in the congregation knew of my surgery, and many would thank me for the example I did not realize I was setting.

The Engineer

With the driving restrictions and recovery expected to take several weeks, arrangements were made for me to work from home. Trying to do anything on the computer seemed impossible, for I could not remember how to log in or access the required files and documents. The plan was for me to take four to six weeks off; however, my associates would call to check on me. The reality of my recovery came as we started to talk about specific projects.

It had been four weeks since surgery when the details of a stressful project were discussed—the Access Control Program and the barrier systems. I could not find the basic names of the equipment we were installing, such as *gate, crash arm*, or *bollard*. I could recall the topic being discussed, but none of the specifics. My head began to ache as the fear of never being able to recover set in.

Fortunately, the people I was associating with knew about my surgery. The program we were discussing was very stressful, and the person who filled in for me struggled with the documentation of cancelling the projects. Seems this project was jinxed, for within six months he had a grand mal seizure. The cause of the seizure was stress and not taking appropriate care of his physical needs.

When I returned to the office, everyone thought I could resume my role as a project manager and work on the projects assigned to me before surgery. When I started reviewing one of the contracts with the Access Control Program, my brain went crazy. I was inundated with a sense of fear that caused a panic attack, and I could not continue to work. As the aura started, I closed the file and threw it back into the file drawer. As the drawer closed, the aura subsided and went away.

My brain seemed unable to comprehend the details of the emails I received concerning other projects. Writing responses was difficult, and remembering who to call and where to go seemed impossible to remember. After several weeks, I went to see Bruce, a friend who now worked in an upper management position. We had worked together on several projects, and he was aware of my abilities prior to surgery. Now I needed guidance on how to inform management that I could no longer perform the work I once excelled at. As we discussed some of the projects we had worked on, he began to realize my ability to recall the details was severely impacted and recommended I write a letter about what happened and my expectations.

The letter should have taken less than an hour to write and now required nearly a day to assemble and arrange the words to make sense. Even then, the grammar and format was poor, with repetitiveness and incorrect punctuation. A few days later, I presented the letter:

Subject: Jon Sadler's Request and Safety Issues

I have been epileptic for nearly 30 years. The problem was handled well with medication until last year, when I started having more seizures than usual having been through several types of medication. I was able to keep things under control however my medication was so high I started having reactions to the medication.

John's Hopkins recommended surgery. The surgery took place on 15 May 2006. Due to some issues with my memory I was to undergo some additional testing in July. All went well. My medications have been reduced, with further reduction scheduled this fall (with a plan to possibly take me off all medications that I have been on for nearly 30 years).

I continued to have some kind of reaction that was not explained to me until last week. Call me the "Air-Head" for during the surgery a bubble was left in my head.[11] It caused dizziness after physical activity or excitedness.

My preference is to stay away from the PM (project management) effort for a couple of months till my thought processes are tested. As I have explained to others I have had the file cabinets in my head rearranged, including some of the doors locked, walkways damaged and ladders removed. I have found alternate ways to get to the file cabinets and have gotten faster at doing so (the ones with the spider webs don't function due to age not surgery). However work is going to help fix this and if I can do some writing etc. let me loose. My driving will return in a few weeks, however it has been over a year since I have driven on any highways and I will need some "training" time before I take off again down I-95.

I have never let epilepsy control my life. I have been physically active and have a family. For work I was the waterfront/utilities specialist for the Navy, budget and cost tracking for a Contractor and you know the story for the Army Corps. I've looked for ways to help Hopkins, for the surgery is only 5 years old and I am the first engineer to go through the(ir) process.

Your assistance on this matter is appreciated. If necessary I will take a pay cut or GS level reduction due to the PM issue.

Sincerely,
Jon Sadler

---

[11] This was an example of my memory issues. The air bubble had to be repeated to me several times after surgery and follow-up doctor appointments.

Bruce took action the next day and went to see Jerry in contracting division. Jerry had a project that needed special attention, and he did not have the staff. It was perfect for me in recovering my math and organizational skills. It involved evaluating close to four hundred contract modifications. It took me days to organize the documents and weeks to evaluate the numbers. I was transposing numbers and could not remember more than three numerals at a time. It would take extra time for me to evaluate the changes. Yet as I worked more and more, my abilities seemed to improve. My review took over three months to perform. My presentation of the materials was clear and concise. Based on the information, the government recovered a large sum of money for overcharges by a contractor. I felt great for my ability to process numbers was back, and I was able to more than pay for my own salary several times over. I could be a project manager again.

Setback

Bruce had another assignment for me involving a presentation to a local chapter of the military engineers. It was a slide presentation with notes to be read on each slide. The session went very well, and I felt great even though I had a couple of auras just before and during the session. Many of the members wanted to talk after the presentation, and I was having difficulty responding for I could not find the information in my brain. Fortunately, I had to leave for an appointment at Johns Hopkins.

My neurologist was not available, and I met with the surgeon. He got excited (and maybe frustrated) when I told him about my auras. He explained how they determined how much of my hippocampus to remove and now wished they had taken out a little more. The autopsy indicated the section of my brain removed was hardened, indicating severe damage.

An EEG was ordered, and I was to wait thirty minutes in the exam room before heading to the test location. Depending on the outcome, we would talk about having surgery again and other techniques available to remove more of the hippocampus. Inside I was broken. It seemed impossible to go through what happened the first time again. The surgeon told me to wait in the exam room and in a few minutes, he would walk with me to where the EEG would be performed. When he returned, he apologized, for the EEG could not be done for a few hours, and I would have to wait out in the waiting area.

I walked into the waiting area and sat down, fighting back tears as my emotions went rampant. To go through what I had previously experienced, especially on my own, made the thought of all the pretest and surgery unbearable. Finally, I decided it was not worth going through all this again. Walking back to the receptionist was difficult and scary. The surgeon was available, and I was told to wait by the desk. When he came out, I said, "I cannot go through this again. I'm leaving now." He was disappointed and started to talk about how the EEG would be good for me to pursue. Emotionally, I was torn apart, for in the morning there was the presentation I helped with where I was speaking in front of more than fifty people and was complimented on my knowledge and abilities. An hour later, I was back to having to deal with my biggest fear: if surgery was performed again, who would I be when it was over?

The Child with Cerebral Palsy

As I waited for the elevator, there were three other people standing near me. Each one of us had been told something about our health that seemed to be a major setback. We made eye contact as we waited and said nothing, for we were engrossed in our own grief. The elevator seemed to take forever to arrive, and when the doors opened, we quickly walked in. In the sixty seconds it would take to get to the ground floor, we were all changed by a child suffering from severe cerebral palsy.

She was about twelve years old and in a special wheelchair where she could lay back so her body could straighten. She was completely immobile as her fingers, arms, legs, and head never moved. The only part of her body that appeared to move was her mouth and eyes as she looked at each person individually. When her eyes locked in with each of us, she smiled. When she smiled, her entire face lit up. As this happened to each of us, we smiled back, and then we could not stop smiling.

When the elevator arrived at the ground floor, we thanked the girl and her mother for the experience as we walked off. The young lady did the only thing she could—she smiled back. Her mother smiled but could not say anything as she was crying too. She had just witnessed how her quadriplegic daughter was able to help each of us to see our situations in a better way. As the doors closed to take them to their floor, we saw the mother wipe away her own tears. The four of us then took a moment to reflect and share the effect the young lady had on each of us. Her actions were such an uplift in our spirits that we could now take on the challenges that each of us faced with hope.

First Grand Mal

It had been six months since the surgery, and everything seemed to be getting better. I was very excited to buy a car and be able to drive again. This time I made sure the vehicle had a manual transmission and the emergency brake on the center console in case I had a seizure while driving. With a manual transmission, the car will stall if my foot is not on the gas pedal or if someone pulls the emergency brake hard. Worst case, they can push hard on the gearshift and place it into neutral. It would not be the best thing for the transmission, but who cares when someone's life may be at risk?

My confidence was shaken soon after getting the car and going on a trip with my family to see my sister Susan in North Carolina. This was the first road trip since surgery. When we arrived at her home, my nephew was curious about what had happened and wanted to talk about my surgery. As we talked, my anxiety level increased, and I was getting concerned about having a seizure. I tried to change the subject; however, he was curious and kept asking questions about the procedure and recovery. He did not realize what was happening and my need to stop thinking about the most traumatic event in my life. I started to have an aura and managed to get it to stop when I walked away from him. Late that night, I had a grand mal seizure in my sleep.

Susan called her friend who was a paramedic; he lived a few minutes away. He notified the ambulance team and rushed over to her house. When he arrived, he saw me lying on my side on the floor near the bed I was sleeping in, and he administered oxygen to help me recover. My body was partially blue from the breathing being interrupted by the seizure. The ambulance team arrived and talked to Wes, who I could see was pulling information about my medications from my wallet and talking to a paramedic. Upon seeing my color return and learning of my seizure history, it was agreed I did not require any further medical assistance. I quickly fell back to sleep and slept until the middle of the morning when everyone was up and planning for the day.

There was a change in my recovery this time. In lieu of my cognitive abilities taking two to three days to recover, it now took a couple of hours. Recovery of the muscle groups involved still required several days. Initially, I was upset for this was quite a setback. I reminded myself my brain was still healing/recovering from surgery. After breakfast, the boys started to play catch football, so I went outside and joined them. The paramedic came by later that morning and was surprised to learn I was out hiking with my children. He was amazed to see how well I was doing in such a short period of time.

Extensive problem-solving, not sleeping eight to ten hours a day, and talking about seizures were the healers and the triggers to the seizures. Putting the mind to work required mapping new ways to store and retrieve information. Being motivated through other people was crucial. I started to cross paths with other people dealing with epilepsy and other disabilities. Surgery changed my life, just in an unexpected way, and not like I had feared. I could crawl out of my shield of hiding and be more open about living with epilepsy.

Second Grand Mal Seizure

My sons were still active in scouting, and a trip to the Boy Scouts High Adventure Camp in Philmont, New Mexico, was being discussed. Adult leaders were needed to participate. The trip was not to occur for a couple of years and would give me time to recover from my surgery. Within a few months, the trip was moved up the following year—less than a year away and just over a year after having surgery. I was so excited I signed up to be one of the adults to go with them.

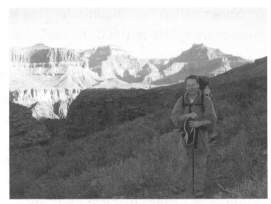

When a friend from church heard about my endeavors, he invited me to hike to the bottom of the Grand Canyon with himself, his son, and a friend of his son's. It would be an incredible journey requiring five days of backpacking to the Colorado River at the bottom of the canyon, just over five thousand feet in elevation. We would be going in late March—four months before the trip to Philmont. It seemed like a wonderful plan to help me get back in shape and regain confidence in myself; I immediately accepted.

I freaked out when we arrived and saw the size and magnitude of the canyon. As we walked along the ridge, I was having ten to twelve auras an hour. Going down into the canyon meant isolation, for cell phones do not work past the first few hundred feet. I was giving serious consideration to getting a hotel room to stay in as the others went on the hike. Then I told everyone about my seizures, and they were fine with my going with them. My confidence was restored, and the next morning, we started the five- day hike in the canyon.

I could not believe this was happening. And once my fear of seizures and falling was under control, I was amazed at what I could do. Several times an hour, my cohorts heard me say, "This is incredible." I said it so often they asked if I could start using some other words like *amazing* or *awesome*. I continued with *incredible*, for I never imagined I could ever do this, ever!

Eventually, we came to a section of the trail where there had been a rockslide and the trail was wiped out. To get through, we had to hang on to a boulder and inch our way around it with a three-hundred-foot drop along the ledge we were on. As I came around, I could feel the weight of my pack pulling me away from the bolder toward the abyss behind me. Fortunately, about the time I was going to slip away, I stepped onto the trail on the other side. My knees were shaking, yet I had no auras. It was an incredible journey, and I was capable of doing it!

Over the next five days, we saw some of the most beautiful sites in the world and climbed along narrow pathways with no safety rails and drop-offs of several hundred feet. At the bottom of the canyon are beautiful beaches of pure white sand with the roar of the Colorado River reflecting off the canyon walls. I got over my fear of heights and stood along a ridge with a three-thousand-foot drop-off to peer down at the river below. During this time, I had no auras or seizures, and I would not have any problems until I came home, where the change in the environment and elevation triggered some auras.

I was most vulnerable to having a seizure during the first twenty-four hours of traveling to a new location.[12] I was feeling good about being able to go to Philmont with the boys. Three weeks prior to the trip, we went to Ocean City. Early the next morning, while asleep, I was awakened by an aura. I walked around the house we were renting and felt exhausted. I returned to the bed and fell right back to sleep. Within an hour, I was reawakened by another aura. This one was much more intense. As I tried to get out of the bed, I fell and hit my head on the edge of the nightstand. I lay on the floor and could not move. I could see the side of the bed but could not hear anything.

My wife got up and, seeing me on the floor, called 911. It was early Sunday morning when this was happening, and the assumption

---

[12] This is related to the seizure trigger "change in environment."

made by the paramedics and the hospital staff was I was having a reaction to a drug overdose. I could not move or speak as I was transported to the hospital. Just as we were turning into the drive to the ER of the hospital, I could finally tell the paramedic my name.

I told the doctor about my surgery a year before, and they ordered a CAT scan. Upon seeing it, they believed everything I said. They could see the forward third of my left temporal had been removed, and a tunnel existed where my hippocampus used to be. They immediately determined I was telling the truth about the seizures and epilepsy, and no further observation or testing involving misuse of drugs was necessary.

I asked if I could be given some ice for my eye that was swelling shut from hitting the corner of the night table. A few hours later, I was feeling better and was discharged. As I was getting ready to leave, I asked for a copy of the CAT scan to give to my neurologist. When I got home, I viewed it on my computer. And for the first time, I saw how much of my brain had been removed. I was shocked. In a side view, I could see four circular plates. Each had five tabs with screws going into my skull. In the back of where the skull had been removed were two nails, about an inch long. The cross section views showed a cavern where the forward section of the temporal lobe had been removed, providing access to the hippocampus. A path or hole could be seen where the hippocampus used to be.

A few years later, when I saw the movie *Master and Commander*, there is a scene where a doctor in the early 1800s does brain surgery on a member of the crew. The patient was suffering from a severe concussion and was in a coma. The doctor drilled a hole through his skull to relieve the pressure, then he placed a five-pound gold piece over the opening and nailed it in place. I complained to my friends that all I got was four quarters, twenty screws, and two nails. Everyone laughed.

When we returned home from our vacation, I was prepared to fight with the staff at Philmont about being allowed to participate in the ten-day hike. Their policy was no one could participate if they had a seizure within the last six months. Just before I made the call,

Wesley came to me and shared his concern. He had seen me have many seizures. In the last two, he played a major role with getting the appropriate medical assistance I needed. He told me how he would not be able to sleep or go too far away from me during the trip for fear of my having a seizure. He saved my life more than once, so I listened to him. He made me aware that I had to consider how my seizures affected my family, not just me. Within a week, the scouts found someone to take my place. I was heartbroken because I could not be with my sons. Philmont played a significant role in my life through my scouting trip in 1976. Now my seizures kept me from being there with my boys.

My manner of treating my depression while they were away was to apply my engineering and construction skills and build a patio on the back of our house. My energy to carry the brick and dig out the area came from the anger inside me. I had no problem getting the soil beneath the brick compacted as I pounded the dirt and cried several times during the days it took to place the brick. I was angry at God, society, the Boy Scouts, and myself.

Reading Skills Improving

My reading skills were improving, and there were several books on how people overcame the fear of seizures and studies on how the brain works. Jill Bolte Taylor had just published *A Stroke of Insight*. Jill is a neuroscientist who suffered a stroke and had surgery similar to mine in the area of her left temporal lobe and hippocampus. The first part of the book is about her having a stroke, which has some similarities to a seizure. To improve my memory, I highlighted the parts I found most applicable to myself. I highlighted over half of the text in the section on recovery. Jill did well with what she planned and worked on. When something changed, she had difficulty remembering and adjusting. The most difficult part was how her brain required eight years of recovery. For myself, it would take ten years. In fact, I continue to recover as I discover more about myself and my abilities.

The most important part I learned from the book is that recovery will only continue if there is a need for the brain to do so. If there is no desire and need, the brain will not adjust and will acclimate. If there is a demand, the brain will find ways to make it happen. We have over a trillion neurons that make up our brains. They rewire and strive to find new manners of connecting when there is a requirement to make it happen.

Chapter 11

Overcoming Disabilities

I brought up the coping mechanism to some people lately. Talked about just accepting your issue and moving on, instead of WOE IS ME. I used our morning laugh sessions with Steve. You were the half-wit, I had no leg to stand on, and Steve (lazy eye) stared at, I dunno. But to me it's still a good object lesson of when beaten down, LAUGH. So, if the Right Hemisphere was itching, it was ME, PEG LEG.
—A text to me from Rick after one of his group sessions with people dealing with amputation

The people at the army corps were helping me with and believing in my recovery. After completing the review of all the change orders, Bruce reviewed my recovery with me and said he had a team working on cleaning up ordnances and an oil spill at a site and needed my help. The site had been used for testing mines (explosives) up through the Vietnam War. It was a large area being prepared for placement of a facility associated with the latest Base Realignment and Closure program. The contract was awarded at $8 million, and the work had just started.

We did not know the amount of the materials involved in the cleanup, and the contract was based on actual cost the contractor had in performing the work. As more and more of the area was surveyed and materials uncovered, more men and equipment was required, and the cost increased. The field team called every day to report finding another area with buried waste that required cleanup. Within twelve months, the project had grown to over $22 million. I took on the role of project manager and coordinated with the post the costs incurred to obtain the funds required to complete the work.

My biggest challenge was reversing the digits in the numbers as I entered them into a computer or wrote them down. For example, $1,250,750 would be clear in my mind yet written as $1,520,750. To say the least, this caused a fair amount of confusion as the totals were never correct. Even when I reviewed the numbers over and over, there were some I left reversed. The best technique for checking the numbers came from my work associate. He was partially dyslexic, and his biggest challenge was arranging words properly in the reports he wrote. To correct this, he read out loud what he was writing. The computer took care of the spelling and punctuation issues.

Initially, I found this very annoying and asked why he had to do it. He explained how reading out loud enabled him to recognize the order of the words being out of place or a word missing in his sentence. Once l learned this, he went from being annoying to be a motivator. I applied the technique for myself and could verify the numbers and correct them as necessary.

The project was completed within a year. Management had me move to a section into the construction division responsible for evaluating contract proposals. This would be a major challenge to my brain for the evaluations were on multimillion dollar projects and were very extensive and detailed. Reports ranged from 30 to 150 pages. This was where Rick worked. And when he learned I would be working with him, he was relieved. He remembered the day we looked at each other and laughed over our situations and upcoming surgeries.

There was another person nearby who had a wandering eye known as strabismus. Each morning, the three of us would get together and talk about the challenges we faced. Then we would help one another understand ourselves and, most importantly, laugh. We came up with nicknames. Rick was known as A Leg Less, or simply Legless (now Peg Leg). The associate with strabismus was referred to as "Are you looking at me?" With a section of my brain missing, I was known as the Half-wit. To this day, Rick and I refer to each other as Peg Leg and the Half-wit.

Chapter 12

Exposure

People with disabilities have the ability to not be disabled.

First Counselor

It had been nearly three years since my surgery. To help with my adjustment and recovery, I tried to find a counselor who could understand what I was going through. My first counselor worked in a room where she dimmed the lights and had a background noise I found uncomfortable. She seemed to be overwhelmed with what I wanted to talk about and just "ooohd" and "awed" in her responses. Within twenty minutes, I had an aura and had to leave. This was totally worthless and not helpful at all. It took a couple of years before I found a counselor who helped guide me to apply my experience and reach out to others.

In Front of the Crowd

Wes and Steve were in a competition band at their high school, and I volunteered to be on the pit crew team to build and bring the backdrops on and off the field. The competition involved high school bands consisting of sixty to one hundred students that performed on the football fields at schools from all over the region. Travel could take up to two hours in each direction. The competitions took place on Saturday evenings, and it was not unusual to get home after midnight. I figured it would be good exposure to people and crowds to help in overcoming my fears. Most importantly, it was a way for me to be with my boys.

Nearly twenty parents volunteered to be on the pit crew as we had approximately five minutes to set up the field displays for the band and three minutes to take it down. The backdrops were twelve-by-eight-inch pictures of the New York skyline. It was fun to unload all the equipment, watch the boys prepare for the competition, and help with getting the equipment on the field. Being on the field scared me, especially in such a large crowd in the stands. It was also very helpful as it helped me defeat my fear of exposure to people and make some new friends through the parent group.

The second year, the theme was "Fear." There were ten four-by-ten-inch banners with the titles to various types of fear. The one I closely related to was agoraphobia—the fear of everything. The band did very well again and was invited to play in a Disney World parade. My exposure on and off the field reinforced my ability to participate and work with other people. Little did I know at the time the significance of the trip to Disney World. Not only did we get to see the parade but the parents also got to see the boys play in concerts and enjoy the rides. My ability to travel and participate in the rides provided hope to another family dealing with seizures.

The Young Man with Spina Bifida

One of the members of the band suffered with spina bifida, and I was amazed to see how far he had come in his life. I remembered my brother, when working on his doctorate in the 1970s, spent time with children suffering from spina bifida. During that time, it was unusual for a child to live beyond five years of age. Through research, they found manners of treating the condition. Now here was a sixteen-year-old boy, a straight A student, who did not let his condition stop him from participating in the band and other school activities. He never thought of himself as disabled.

He played a keyboard, so the pit crew built a platform for him to sit on and play. The band members liked to be around him. And on the days he got tired of being in his wheelchair, he would sit on the floor in the band room. When he did this, everyone else in the band would sit down on the floor too. On the day of graduation, I walked up to him and thanked him for being such an inspiration to me. Seeing his abilities helped me conquer my fears of being in public and inspired me to push beyond my limits to help my brain recover—to demand it "rewire."

Chapter 13

The Calling (2009–2010)

His son was four years old and had intractable seizures.

Sharing Experience

It had been three and a half years since my surgery. My memory was improving, and my confidence was building. There was a gentleman I met through work who, learning of my having epilepsy, wanted to see me. He had been having seizures most of his life and needed to talk to someone who could relate to what he was dealing with.

He came into my office, introduced himself, and asked if I had a minute to talk. As he sat down, he told me about learning of my having brain surgery for my seizures and wanted to share what it had been like for him to live with epilepsy. He had an amazing positive attitude about living with seizures. Like many people dealing with seizures, he never had a driver's license and relied on public transportation. He shared his story of how his attitude changed from feeling guilty and depressed about his dependency on others to feeling fulfilled.

We both had relied on other people for transportation; his sources came through a church he attended. The dependency on other people for transportation provided a manner for those people to apply their God-given talents and gifts. I had witnessed this many times through the support from my church, and now I realized how my dependency was one of God's tools in inspiring others. It is amazing how a difficult situation can give a person a new perspective on themselves, especially when the situation makes a person feel hopeless. Having this new perspective made me wonder even more about my situation and what my calling was. The old question came back to me again: "What am I in training for?" How was I supposed to work with other people when I was so humiliated, embarrassed, and fearful of the repercussions caused by a seizure?

The Phone Call

A few months later came a phone call from a gentleman in association with my work in construction. We were discussing our availability to review the technical requirements of a contract. He told me he could not meet the following week for he had a family conflict. He was dedicated to his job; however, his priority was to take his son on a Make-A-Wish trip to Disney World. I assured him this would not be a problem and continued to talk about another time that may work for us. It was then the father said, "We received the grant from the Make-A-Wish foundation for my child has epilepsy."

For me, the world came to a standstill. This could not be happening. Should I share my own experience or keep quiet? If I share it, will he doubt me and think less of me? For nearly a minute, there was complete silence as I debated in my mind what to say. I decided it was not important for this person to know of my condition. Besides, if his child is going on a Make-A-Wish trip, my experience should not be important.

With the phone being silent for so long, the person thought I had hung up or the phone had failed. He was about to hang up and call me back when I responded, "Your son and I have much in common."

Suddenly, our discussion changed from work to epilepsy. I shared part of my story—of being treated for nearly thirty years with medication and having a lobectomy, affecting the left temporal lobe of my brain. About every five minutes, I was interrupted as he said, "But you're a project manager," as he could not believe someone with epilepsy and brain surgery could achieve so much.

It had been less than a year since I had been to Disney World on the band trip with my wife and children. We rode several rollercoasters and seen many shows. It was a wonderful time, for everyone in the family got to be a child again, and we got to watch our children perform and march in the parade. I talked of riding the rollercoasters and going to the shows. It had been nearly two hours since we started talking, I had never shared so much of my own experience with someone I had never met, and I was totally exhausted. Little did I realize how my experience influenced the person.

A few weeks later, we had our meeting, and one of the fellow's coworkers and close friend asked if he could talk to me in private. We went into another room and sat down. The gentleman started by thanking me for being open about my epilepsy and how everyone now had hope that people with epilepsy have a future. I fought back tears and had difficulty thanking the man for sharing this information. I was overwhelmed. This was the explanation to my living longer than the twenty years I had in my contract with God. It was God's way of telling me to reach out with my experience and provide hope to those sharing similar experiences.

Answering the Call

A whole new part of my life was coming together. I stopped by the office of the local Epilepsy Foundation, Chesapeake Region, Towson, Maryland. I had seen the sign many times over the past five years as my sons were going to school nearby.

Here I met Mary Wontrop, the director of the chapter, and expressed my interest in being involved. Within a few weeks, she told me of the HOPE mentoring program the Epilepsy Foundation has for people to be mentors[13]. The acronym HOPE stands for "Helping Other People with Epilepsy." Within two months, I received the training and started doing something I never thought I should or could do—sharing my story with more and more people. This would

---

[13]   H.O.P.E. is a trademark of UCB, Inc., Atlanta, Georgia, for its epilepsy mentoring program, licensed by the Epilepsy Foundation and its local chapters' use.

change from sharing my story to simply applying my experience to be an effective counselor for people with seizure disorders.

Applying the Call

I found a mental health counselor who could relate in some ways with me, for he had situations in his life that he had struggled through too. Although he could not relate with my recovery, he helped with family and relationship issues. When I told him what was happening with the people I met, the work I was doing with my church, the epilepsy foundation, and my motivation to recover, he asked me about going to graduate school. In some ways, I thought he was crazy. I could never do that with the way my brain functioned.

As he learned more about my motivational skills and my life experiences, he again suggested I considered becoming a counselor. This time he was more specific and suggested becoming a pastoral counselor—a program offered by Loyola University in Baltimore, Maryland. As I learned more about the program, the more excited and concerned I became. The questions that laced me with doubt were "How is a person, who can't remember names, ever going to get through the studies and the exams associated with courses I would have to take?" The other question being "How would I coordinate working full time, attend classes, and complete all the work assignments?" Yet everything seemed to be coming together for me to do the program.

I did the interviews, handed in my application, and was accepted into the program. With an engineering degree, I did not have any of the criteria completed. I would go through all the prerequisites for the two-year internship and finish the remaining courses required to graduate. I was moving forward totally on a spiritual calling. My brain could not conceive of being able to work well enough to complete twenty-two courses on a subject matter I had never studied before.

Section 6

Recovery and Graduate School

Chapter 14

Graduate Degree in Pastoral Counseling (2010–2015)

Though my body appears whole, the operation and
control center of my brain is damaged. It can only be
fixed by a demand to rewire . . . work with me.

Although Loyola University was founded by a Jesuit priest in 1852, the pastoral counseling program did not focus on a particular religion or faith. The students, instructors, and professors were of different backgrounds, faiths, and religions. Some people were not associated with any religion yet had a strong spiritual connection with God. Still others were priests, chaplains, or pastors. Most of us were on a second or third career and felt a calling through experience to provide support to others. Unlike other counseling programs, the studies and discussions were expanded to include how God and prayer are important in every person's life. Appropriate application of a spiritual nature was reviewed throughout the classes and internships required to help us grow and develop into effective counselors.

Most classes started with a classmate talking about an experience, or sharing a part of a book or poem, that helped them grow in understanding how God works through people and is ever present. Many courses consisted of people of various Protestant, Catholic, Hindu, Buddhist, and Islamic faiths. People with disabilities were given the support they needed in the classes, either by other students or the disability programs provided by the university.

A majority of the students were working full time and planned on completing the program in three to seven years. The master's degree included studies in humanities, statistics, religion, ethics, and law. In addition, we studied individual, family, and group counseling, social and racial issues, and theories and techniques to apply in various settings. Four of the courses taught how to develop individual techniques during an internship in clinical work. To work full-time and complete the program was quite a challenge for anyone. My hopes of completing the program were crushed after a few weeks of classes. Then came the realization that the "impossible is possible" as the program proved to be the best treatment to enable my brain to recover from surgery and the damage caused by my head injuries and seizures.

The clinical courses involved working in a counseling facility eight to twenty hours per week, along with additional supervision hours, writing extensive papers, and attending weekly classes. A total of eight hundred hours of clinical work, including 280 hours of one-on-one counseling with clients, was required for graduation. To assure the interns understood the roles of a counselor, they had to have experience being the client. If interns had not seen a counselor before, they were required to do so for an extensive period of time in order to fully comprehend what was taught in the classes.

Failure or Reaching Out?

Through the requirements of each course and the people involved came numerous lessons about humility and witnessing survival and perseverance through faith. Several colleagues had experienced traumatic events, and others had disabilities that impaired their learning in a typical class setting. I was humbled, yet I witnessed and developed manners on how to ask others for support. In my first semester, I took a course on humanities taught by Professor Frank Richardson. I had told a fellow student who sat next to me about my epilepsy and what to do if I had a seizure. She was curious and asked more questions, so I told her about my surgery and disability. She was fascinated by how far I had come in recovery and played a key role in my getting through the program.

Four weeks later, we had our first exam. The format of the exam was relatively simple: just fill in the blank at the end of the question.

It was frustrating that the first letter of the word required to answers the question would come to my mind, but I could not recover the entire word. When our graded exams were returned, I had less than 50 percent marked on the side, with an F written at the top of the front page. My classmate saw this and asked me if I was going to talk to the professor about my disability. I said no because my hopes were gone, and I figured I would eventually fail out of the entire program. She looked straight at me and told me, "After class, you have got to tell the professor about your disability. If you do not, I will." She made sure I did not abscond and escorted me to the front of the classroom to see the professor. I was about to be taught the greatest lesson on the power of humility.

There were several people ahead of me waiting to speak to the professor, and I just wanted to leave. However, my classmate stayed and talked about the importance of sharing my experience and asking for support. For me, this was one of those humiliating times for I had never required disability services in a class before. Professor Richardson was a quiet, easygoing person who was vested in getting us through the program. He was an ordained pastor, with a PhD in psychology and many years' experience working with people with disabilities. As I approached him, I felt despondent knowing I would never be able to get better grades with my brain injury. He looked at me and said, "It is good you came to talk to me for I needed to know what happened on the exam." I did not know what to say, so my friend promptly told him that I needed special assistance on taking exams. Of course, the professor's response was "Why?"

Declaring Disability

When I told him about my epilepsy and surgery, he asked me, "What is required for you to pass an exam?" I replied, "I need a list of words, and please do not give me the standard *A B C D* form of answering system. Just provide a list of nine to twelve words somewhere on the page, and I will know which is correct. I also need additional time to take an exam. If this can be arranged, it would be very helpful." He got very excited as he explained to me why I should have told him about this sooner. I was surprised; he was not only willing to work with me, but it was also important to him to do so. He went on to explain that the exam we had just taken would not be counted in my final grade. In addition, he told me about the program the university has for students with disabilities and how I needed to talk to them right away.

On the next exam, I earned a B. And for everyone in the class, there was a list of nine to ten words after each question. It was incredible, for after reading the question, the first letter to the answer came to my mind. As I reviewed the words provided, I could recognize the correct word, even if several of the words started with the same letter. I usually had to read the problem several times to fully comprehend the question.

I quickly learned how nervousness caused my brain to shut down with no comprehension of what the question was about or even what the words in the question mean. I could read each word; however, the context of the question would not formulate in my mind. Staying calm was critical. It would take time and practice to learn how to stay calm and allow my mind to absorb what was happening. I was amazed at how I could recall the answers and pleased I earned a low B to high C grade on every exam. Passing the course was now very possible.

Sometimes the answer would appear in my mind, yet I could not comprehend the importance of it. Prior to surgery, the answer would come to me, and I could remember it for a while as I wrote it down. Now the answer seemed to suddenly appear and then disappear. Often it would never reappear, especially when I got apprehensive or frustrated. This was something that would take time to understand and control.

Preparing for the tests required many hours of study and discovering techniques to recall names and titles. I had difficulty with such things prior to surgery in 2006, as demonstrated in the testing done during the five-day EEG. At that time, I scored in the

34 percentile, meaning 66 percent of the people in my classification scored higher than me. After surgery, my score went to less than one percent, the lowest rating possible. The more I tried to remember something, the less I could recall. Frustration would set in, and everything I was reading and working on would go blank (activating the old path in my mind that was a dead end).

When everyone else finished their exam, the professor would take me to another room, where I would work for another thirty to forty-five minutes. Whenever I got nervous or excited, my brain would use the old path of memory processing and slam into the void in my head and go blank. When I calmed down, the words would flash up and be gone in an instant. Often, I doubted whether the word was correct as the meaning of the word was not there. With time, more than the first letter of the word would appear. Often by writing it down and repeating it, the whole word would appear. My level of intelligence was not impaired by the surgery; it was the ability to recall specific words.

The overall class grade was primarily based on the final paper due at the end of the semester. The paper was to be based on a personal perspective of our lives and how our experience(s) have impacted our life views. My paper was based on living with epilepsy and discovering how to help others persevere through similar challenges. This is when I learned of my professor's interest in working with people with epilepsy, especially his willingness to work with me.

He would not share this until the papers were turned in and graded. It was our last class, and he started by explaining more of his background, the experiences he had as a child, and his ministry. His mother had epilepsy, and as a child, he witnessed her have many grand mal seizures. It was during a time when the ignorance of epilepsy had led to laws limiting a person with epilepsy to be educated and marry in many states. He talked of his mother having a very long seizure while on a road trip. His siblings had to make room in the car for her to lie down and recover. He found a spiritual connection that helped him survive and thrive in working with other people—first through the church and later as a psychologist. He worked with many people dealing with disabilities throughout his career.

At the end of class, he handed back our papers. I saw the number 498 on the top of the front page, and my mouth fell open in shock. This was 498 points out of 500. On the second page was an A and a note about how he related to my experience. He assured me I could work through the program and wished me the best in my efforts. I was so amazed at how well I did on the paper and the influence epilepsy had on the professor. I had tears streaming down my face.

Learning How to Learn

This period of my life required learning how to learn. The simple part was working through the Disabilities Office provided by the university. Upon confirmation of my disability from my neurologist, I was able to obtain special services and notifications provided to my professors of my disability. The special assistance I received was additional time to take my exams and recording classes. This additional time was essential in enabling my brain to search out the answer within my head. It was crucial in controlling nervousness while taking an exam. When this happened, my brain would follow the old passage through my left hippocampus to get to the database where my memory would crash into a dead end. My brain not only had to find and follow the route to the answer but was also being required to develop new patterns for the information to be located and transposed so I could write out the answers. Sections of my brain needed to rewire based on the demand to do so.

There were many tools available for me to apply in working with my disabilities in my classes. My neurologist was impressed with my desire to obtain my master's degree. He provided a letter of certification required by the Disabilities Support Office. Primarily, I needed additional time for exams, which was important in overcoming the delays in my memory recall.

Disability Support

The accommodations of the Disability Support Office were essential in completing my classes. The grades for the next several courses were based on take-home exams or writing a series of papers. Many hours would be required to review the answers and assure the math was done correctly or the paper related and answered the specifics of the question(s). In most cases, the professors were very supportive and worked with me.

There was an excellent writing center for support in writing papers. This was a treasure, for there is quite a difference between how a counselor and an engineer writes. The engineer was used to bullets and going straight to the facts. The counselor needs to express everything in full sentences and explanation, with backup documentation appropriately credited. American Psychological Association (APA) formatting was to be followed, requiring a learning curve for me. I was given websites to learn about properly formatting a document, quoting references, and arranging sentences and paragraphs. Writing was frustrating as a sentence would come together in my mind then be lost before completing the typing. This required several minutes of reviewing the context of what I was attempting to say. The staff at the writing center assisted with proofreading and providing guidance on documentation and format.

A few of the courses, such as statistics, had open-book take-home exams with no time limit. Everyone thought that my background as an engineer would make statistics easy for me. Although statistics has numbers and charts, it is a language in itself. Furthermore, my mathematical processing ability had been severely jarred through my seizures and surgery. I thought this course would be one of the most difficult for me, so I took it in my third semester of studies. I also made sure it was my only class for that semester. As the professor demonstrated various methods and techniques in class, there were three of us he called on the most. One of fellows enjoyed being active in the class, asked many questions, and tried to solve many of the problems presented by the professor. When he got stuck or tired, his response would be, "Ask Sadler." There were many classes where my brain was too tired to register what was being discussed. The professor was available during the week to seek assistance.

I was in my third year and studying psychoanalysis, where the professor could not comprehend my disability because I appeared normal as I actively participated in class discussions. She couldn't believe I had such a disability with word recall. However, on the exams, I did well with the multiple choice and poorly on the fill-in-the-blank questions.

I was fascinated with the class. I fit into the diagnosis of anxiety and mood disorders, schizophrenia, and personality disorders at various stages of my life, especially during recovery from a seizure and brain surgery. Some of these symptoms occurred as a side effect of a medication. The reason I would not be diagnosed in these categories is the fact that the symptoms are caused by a neurological disorder—epilepsy.

I maintained a high C average. To test the professor's assumption, she made some revisions to the final exam. The exam was primarily fill-in-the-blank-type questions, and she refused to provide any support. Questions consisted of several sentences relating to specific methods and applications of a diagnosis. As I read through the questions, I noticed key words that would help me answer other questions throughout the exam. Being the last to finish the exam, the professor and her associate graded it for me. I missed one question. This demonstrated my familiarity with the subject matter and validated my disability to express specific names. She realized I was not making up my disability and gave me an A for the class.

Mental Exhaustion

While I was going to school, I was working full time for the Army Corps of Engineers. There would be those evenings, after a trying day at work or suffering from a lack of sleep, which impacted my memory recall. My memory basically shut off. I was unable to learn or recall the subject matter, even though I was physically functional. When asked a question, I responded with "Sorry, I'm tired and my brain is not here." My brain was tired and trying to function through the old paths to my memory. When this happened, it would hit a dead end, literally the void in my head. There were many people in the class who were dealing with memory issue; however, they did not remember for they were bored or could not comprehend the material being taught.

It was difficult to take notes because I could not remember what was said long enough to write it down. I could not write as fast as the professor spoke, and my short-term memory would blank out or would mix the words out of order. I would start a sentence then have no memory of the key words or names affiliated with what I was writing about. My best was writing four words in the start of a sentence; there were many uncompleted sentences in my notes. Fortunately, this was simplified as my poor note-taking skills were offset by the age of electronics.

Electronic Tools

Most of the professors had no problem with the class being recorded by a student with the understanding the recordings were solely for the individual and would be deleted upon completion of the course. In most of my classes, I would record them using my cell phone. I would write down a key word and the time of the recording for cross-referencing. It was not unusual for me to spend several hours each week listening to the recordings and completing my notes.

At the end of my second year, Moodle was implemented by the university. Moodle is a website that enables a student to keep track of their assignments, schedules, and grades. Most importantly, it enabled students to interact with each other electronically and watch recordings of the classes. My stress level dropped as I learned to apply these tools and overcome memory issues. I could listen and see more of what was happening during class and, with practice, access my memory as I listened to the recordings.

It would take three years to reach the stage of having complete notes at the end of class. My brain was working extra hard and exercised through replaying the recordings of the classes over and over. This brought a lot of relief, for such tools helped me overcome memory issues and listen and see more of what was happening during class.

Another very useful tool I discovered was Kindle. Kindle provides an electronic version of the textbook with important features that are especially helpful for people with learning disabilities. Taking notes required highlighting the text and labeling the note to electronically save it. I needed to develop a skill to identify what was important and labeled it. Then I could access the information through the Kindle program on my computer by going to the notes screen and determine what was most applicable to the assignment. These notes were electronically copied and pasted into Word files to assist with my studies and papers.

To help in organizing and writing papers, I discovered the Dragon NaturallySpeaking program. I talked to my computer, and the words would appear on the screen. I was no longer dealing with the delay of typing and the loss of the thoughts.

Inspiration

I had been careful of letting people know I had epilepsy for fear of how they would react and continue to associate with me. Then during my fifth semester, a paper was due, and I was exhausted from the late nights of research, writing, and engineering work earlier in the day. My anxiety level was very high, and the person sitting next to me saw my hands shaking slightly. I was having a partial seizure and had felt an aura come as a wave of nausea passed through me; however, I did not lose consciousness. She asked me if I needed help, and I responded, "No." A few minutes later, I told her about my epilepsy, and she became quiet. Afterward, she sat far away from me in the remaining classes. She would not respond when I tried to get her attention or said, "Hi."

When I started the next semester, I met another student named Curtis, a pastor who was studying for his pastoral counseling degree. On the opening day of every course, we would take a few minutes to learn about the person next to us and then introduce them to the entire class. Curtis seemed like someone I could trust in talking about my epilepsy. I told him about my family, work experience, where I was in the program, and motivation to become a counselor. I also told him about my seizures. Curtis told me about his background, motivation, and calling to work in the pastoral field for me to share when I introduced him. After I introduced Curtis, he introduced me to the class. The first thing he said to everyone was "This is Jon Sadler, and he has epilepsy." He did not intend to mock me for he was fascinated by my motivational and spiritual gifts.

I felt so crushed and so small that the only way to look was up. Everyone in the class now knew of my condition and why they should be afraid of me, or so I thought. Then I realized I had nothing to fear. Everyone knew of my seizure disorder, and I did not have to worry about how they would respond if they saw me have a seizure. In that moment, I felt taller than I ever had, and the ten-thousand-pound weight of dread I carried was gone. I no longer had to hide my disability.

After class, I felt even more inspired, and I fully understood my calling. Three classmates came to me to ask for help in understanding seizures. One had a close friend who was recently diagnosed with epilepsy, and the other two had family members suffering with depression caused by seizures and medication. Their love for their family was part of what inspired them to become counselors. I did not have to say anything as they simply said, "Thank you for sharing your story and never giving up." They wanted to tell my story to the others to bring them hope through the example I was setting. When I returned to my car, I climbed inside and was overwhelmed with what had just happened. It was one of the *ah-ha* moments when all my experience in living with seizures and the doubt and fear of how others would react had deeper meaning. There were more people inspired by my perseverance than feared my seizures. I cried for a long time before heading home.

Curtis provided another insight concerning relationships. He talked of how we each have a path to follow as we journey through life. Our paths cross with other people. Sometimes it is just for a moment; other times the paths go side by side as we journey together through a period of life. In long-term relationships, the paths run side by side for much of our lives. In other instances, we see a person for just a moment. What we do can have a significant influence in their or our lives. A good example of this was the man who provided the new license plate for me in Rhode Island when my license was reinstated. With Curtis, we would journey together for four months as we studied in the same class and cross paths for a moment many times later.

By being honest about my seizure disorder, more people opened up about their issues. I learned from my classmates about dealing with anxiety, depression, deafness, abuse, addictions, and spirituality, to name a few. The key components in their lives focused on survival and hope. Everyone I talked to was driven by a calling received when they were dealing with a difficult time in their lives. For some, it was living with it, and for others, it was being the witness.

Medical Follow-Up

I kept in touch with Dr. Jason Brandt, the professor of psychiatry and behavioral sciences, director, Division of Medical Psychology and Professor of Neurology at Johns Hopkins University, who was interested in my case and motivated me in my experience in recovery and studies. Most of our communication was through email:

From: Jon Sadler
Sent: Monday, July 23, 2012 4:55 PM
To: Jason Brandt
Subject: Sadler Case

Dr. Brandt,

Thought I should give you an update on how I am proceeding with changing careers. I have completed 9 of 22 classes for my degree in Pastoral Counseling. As you may be aware, the studies involve understanding oneself. Through my volunteer work and studies I have learned more about the self-generated fear of seizures and the significance of being open and willing. The first few classes required writing papers about having epilepsy from a first-person vantage and the last few from a third person perspective. It has been interesting how the discussions in the classes have brought out quite a few people dealing with epilepsy through relations with family and friends.

Five of the classes have had closed book quizzes; those that are multiple choice I do well with, those that are fill in the blank I do not for my difficulty locating the words (in my head). Fortunately, only a piece of the overall grade is based on the quizzes. So far the most difficult class was Psychoanalysis which I had this spring, as we studied the DSM-IV-TR. I could relate in a first-person manner to "Anxiety and Mood Disorders", "Schizophrenia", and "Personality Disorders" through my seizures and side effects of medications. The professor was impressed with my ability to provide insight and awareness about making such diagnosis and the importance of verifying the physical condition of the client, medications, etc. (including talking to a neurologist or neuropsychologist). She watched me take quizzes (fill in the blank) and struggle with word recall (I tried several different manners to memorize terms, etc.). I could write a paper indicating a full comprehension of the situation without additional time (OK I was usually last to finish). For the papers, I had access to the manuals/books and knew where to look. The comprehension is there, accessing title through my mental resources was difficult. The last quiz was written in a manner where the wording of the questions related to nearly all the answers (i.e. wording of question 1 had the answers to question 5). I did very well.

My plan is to start clinicals in January 2013 and finish the program in 2015. This will coincide with my retirement as an engineer. Seems the harder I work the better my brain functions.

Hope all is well,

Jon Sadler

He was very helpful in keeping me motivated. The more I studied, the more I could understand what was happening within my own brain. He responded with this:

Dear Jon,
Thank you for taking the time to write and letting me know about your academic progress. It seems that you have a great deal of insight into how your cognitive system works (i.e., metacognition), and your mental strengths and weaknesses. As long as you continue to capitalize on your strengths and minimize your weaknesses, you should do fine!
Keep up the great work!
Best regards,
Jason Brandt, Ph.D., ABPP(CN)

Professor of Psychiatry & Behavioral Sciences
Director, Division of Medical Psychology
Professor of Neurology
The Johns Hopkins University School of Medicine
600 N. Wolfe Street, Meyer 218
Baltimore, MD 21287-7218

Chapter 15

Clinical Work

Challenges in life enable one to grow and take on the future. A sense of joy develops. Joy brings on the ability to grow in dark times. Hope and faith make all things possible.

For my clinical requirements, I worked with peopled dealing with drug and alcohol addictions and others with brain injury. The brain injury work started as group sessions and was coordinated with a fellow student studying speech therapy. We enjoyed working together. He appreciated my sharing experience with speech impediment associated with seizures and brain surgery. He taught me how a speech therapist would have worked with me had I needed assistance. The work with those with brain injury was fascinating as we learned to work together as a counselor and therapist. Although there were many people interested in participating, the program was cancelled due to transportation issues for those needing care.

Mobility has been the biggest challenge for most people dealing with epilepsy because they often have no transportation to see a counselor. In most cases, when a person has a seizure, the state will suspend their driver's license from thirty days to one year. In some states, the department of transportation provides special services for people with disabilities. This is often limited by county or city that has public transportation. In most cases, the person with a seizure disorder depends on family or friends for transportation.

I work with addicts at the Westminster Rescue Mission in Westminster, Maryland. Many of the clients had comorbid conditions because they struggled with depression and anxiety, which they treated with illegal drugs or alcohol. In many cases, they were addicted to both. My third client was dealing with anxiety, alcoholism, abuse, and epilepsy. There were several clients who were suffering with bipolar disorder, which they self-treated with heroin. I found a commonality with many, especially those with bipolar disorders. There are similarities in what happened during my seizures and what they experience in their manic and especially their depressive episodes. The manic episode was similar to my recovery from a seizure as I felt so good to be alive. My depression came with the speech impediments and inability to totally function for several days as the brain recovered. There was also a change in the brain chemistry caused by taking higher doses of medications. High levels of anxiety were usual as I worried about job impact and reactions of my associates.

My ability to associate with their depression and anxiety gave me a perspective that enabled me to quickly build trusting relationships. For many, it was the first time they talked to someone who fully understood what they were dealing with in their lives. Therapy centered on the cause and events that triggered the addictive behavior. Until the client understood the cause, they had no reason to stay clean. They were motivated through a spiritual connection with God to find meaning in their lives and fulfill his calling.

There was a particular client in his midtwenties who was dealing with bipolar disorder. He told me about another therapist he had seen and how the counselor could not relate to his problem. He then thanked me for working with him because I shared some of my experiences with seizures that correlated with his bipolar disorder. He had never understood what his bipolar disorder was, yet he saw it in his father and was now dealing with it himself. The therapy focused on his realizing why he acted and felt the way he did and discovering meaning to what was happening. The major part came through building a spiritual relationship with God. At the end of the first six months, I had to leave and would not be able to keep in touch with him. He left the mission a few days later and started using heroin again to get his emotions to stabilize.

I did my next round of clinicals at a separate agency and then returned to the mission four months after my previous clinical work there had ended. Within two weeks, the same client was accepted back into the mission. We saw each other in the hallway and both felt a spiritual calling in being together again. I would be his counselor for four more months, and I had the client work on seeking medical assistance from a psychologist.

Soon after starting our clinical sessions again, he told me his favorite scripture reading was from Matthew 19:25: "With God all things are possible." He now understood why his mood changed so drastically in such a short period of time. He no longer felt guilt about who he was as he understood his mood was due to his bipolar disorder caused by brain chemistry. Unfortunately, obtaining appropriate care for bipolar disorder may be difficult for those with no resources or money.

HOPE Instilled

My clients suffering from brain injury were the most challenging for me, as I had moments of reflection of my own experience. Often we inspired one another, for the clients searched for positive reinforcement and someone to process his/her life events. I was blessed with an opportunity to apply everything I learned through my life journey and the refinement as an intern in the pastoral counseling program.

At the end of my fourth year, I met a peer who was dealing with seizures and recovery from brain surgery. She had a section of her left temporal lobe removed and was motivated spiritually to become a counselor. A good part of her concerns focused on having self-confidence to be able to complete the program. She shared how her concerns were appeased as she learned about my ability to complete the courses and desire to progress. I never realized the influence I was having on people as they learned my story. We physically came together for a brief moment, and she helped me discover new meaning in my journey. She graduated six months after I did. Hope is inspired two ways: through the definition of the word itself and the acronyms. The definition for me is this: "There is meaning in what is happening, learn, build, believe, for life can be better." The acronym for me, through the Epilepsy Foundation, was "Helping Other People with Epilepsy." Through my studies and experience, this has been revised to "Helping Other People Everywhere."

Chapter 16

The National Counseling Exam

The impossible is possible.

It was the spring semester of my fifth and final year, and I had completed nineteen of the twenty-two courses, including all my clinical work required to graduate. If everything went as planned, my last class would be completed in the summer semester. The biggest challenge now was the National Counseling Exam, known as the NCE.

The NCE is required in most states to obtain clinical licensing and is often taken as a student has completed or only has a few classes to complete in a counseling program. There were several study guides and a program on CDs used in preparing for the exam. For five months, I listened to the CDs repeatedly and read the study guide several times. It was not unusual for me to miss the same question repeatedly. Due to work and classes, my brain was working hard and becoming stressed. Trying to find time to effectively study for the exam was difficult for it was not worth studying or listening to the CDs when I was tired; my memory of what I would hear or read was shut down.

When the day came to take the exam, I was apprehensive and had to calm down because my brain struggled to follow the old paths—the dead ends to my memory. The exam was difficult, and each question consisted of several examples presented in the study guides I had used. As I read through the first twelve problems, I had no comprehension of the subject matter. My brain was blank, and my anxiety level shot through the roof.

By taking a deep breath and relaxing for a minute, my attitude changed from "I must pass" to "I am learning from the exam, and I can always take it again someday." The anxiety dissipated, and the new paths developed over the past few years reopened in my mind. Suddenly, I knew the answer to the next question and the next and the next.

As I finished the last problem, I felt exhausted both physically and mentally. I chuckled as there was still ten minutes left before having to turn it in. As I thumbed through the answer sheet, checking for problems I hadn't answered, I realized I still had the first twelve questions to complete. I could now find the file in my brain that covered the subject matter associated with most of those questions. The time allotted to complete the exam was four hours. I turned mine in after three hours and fifty-nine minutes. I had one minute to spare! There were many people still working on the exam as I left the room. Now the only unanswered question was "Did I pass?" Seems several of my associates had the same question. As I left the room, I was happy and amazed—happy the exam was over and amazed I had made it this far to be able to take it. Miracles can and do happen.

It was several months before the results of the exam came in the mail. The envelope was thin and contained only one page. In my engineering days, when the one-pager was received for the Professional Engineer exam, it meant you failed. In lieu of reading all the details, I just went to the bottom to see my score. It was lower than I hoped for and thought, *You did your best.* I read through the details, and there in small capital letters, I saw PASSING. Once more, I was in tears. Not long ago I thought this would be impossible. I was reminded that through a strong spiritual faith in God, "all things are possible!"

Chapter 17

Self-Thesis The Storm before the Calm

We often do not appreciate how good life is until after we live through a major life challenge, surrounded by self-doubt. Persevering through such times builds faith and hope for the future.

I was getting more and more excited as I completed my fourth year of studies with only three courses to finish. One of the courses was Family Therapy, taught by Professor Richardson,[14] who guided me through my very first course and inspired me with his experience and faith that I could complete the program and become an effective pastoral counselor. When he asked me if I needed any special assistance taking the exams in the class, I smiled and said no. Four years of intense studies and working full-time as an engineer enabled my brain to develop new ways (rewire) to access the memory. The effort to accomplish my degree required controlling my emotions and practicing over and over the methods to remember criteria. I had to stay calm, not get stressed, then patiently wait for the words appear in my mind. I no longer needed any special assistance when taking an exam, including additional time.

Professor Richardson inspired me to apply my experiences in relating to people with disabilities. He shared, "I just facilitated what was already within you, which was a 'can-do' spirit and a motivation not to give up. I saw that in my mother as well. She did not let her epilepsy slow her down. She persevered and had an amazing, resilient

---

[14]   Professor Richardson taught my first course (humanities) and one of the last (family therapy).

spirit. So witnessing her life, I was ready to encourage you to reach for greater heights when you and I were introduced for the first time."

When the spring semester was over, I had the final course to complete to graduate. The course focused on writing a pastoral reflection paper based on my journey to become a pastoral counselor. What better title could I have chosen then—"Sailing the Course: Meaning in the Storms.". The paper focused on the pilgrimage of my living with epilepsy and recovery from surgery, and how I applied what I learned about myself to develop a professional ability to help other people.

Storms are a metaphor demonstrated how life can be wearisome yet build character; they can make a person strong or break them. Sailing is used as a lens through which to view life events, survival, recovery, and a spiritual calling. The perspective is that of an experienced sailor who has felt a spiritual closeness when under sail. The sailor faces challenges, including the inability to see or control the wind, which is vital to the operation of the boat. Just as rough waters and high winds impact a sailor's capacity to continue to sail, serious life events and tragedy influence a person's strength to find meaning in life, faith, and still have hope for the future.

I was writing about my future with exposure to people dealing with trauma, addictions, and physical and/or brain injuries. The goal was to instill hope and confidence in others as they face the storms they encounter in life. Even before completing the paper, I was about to be tested through a very serious storm.

My brother-in-law, Michael, was in the hospital for open-heart surgery. The surgery was successful, and he was progressing well until there was confusion with his treatment among the staff. Michael had been suffering for over fifteen years with a degenerative spinal condition and required medication for his pain. Some of the staff were not made aware of this and refused to provide the appropriate pain medication. His pain became excruciating. And over the next five days, he suffered three more heart attacks. After the second heart attack, he had met with one of the pastoral staff and found peace within himself and with God. Two days later, he had his third heart attack, slipped into a coma, and was kept in a comatose state by lowering his body temperature in hopes he would recover.

For the next three days, I was with my sister Susan and Michael's family while we waited to see if he would recover from his third heart attack There were late nights where Susan agonized in making tough decisions and suffered with the trauma of having watched the man she loved suffer with severe pain and being brought back to life after his heart stopped time and again. What we did not realize was Michael may have had some cognitive awareness each time his heart stopped and the doctor's worked to revive him. Michael suffered with seeing death over and over.

When I visited Michael in intensive care, I could see the lines of the EEG and knew he was dead, kept alive by machine. I did not share this with anyone. I did well as I worked as a brother, friend, and counselor with the family, yet I broke down several times when alone due to the loss of the brother I loved. After three days, the doctors started to revive Michael by raising his body temperature. As it slowly increased, his body started to tremble and slipped into a grand mal seizure. To stop the seizure, his body temperature was quickly lowered, and he was pronounced dead by the medical staff. My sister Susan and Michael's family were crushed as we watched the hospital staff do their work. The pastoral care unit was outstanding. Michael was given his last rights, and we watched him die as the support systems were turned off. Susan wept little because she was so traumatized by what happened that week. The tears came later. I did not have time to think about what had just happened. That would come later. Right now, I had to complete my paper and graduate.

With Michael, I was exposed to the traumatic loss of a loved one. In the reflection paper, I further expressed how my faith grew during this time by relying on God. The is the same faith that brought me through such trying times and made me spiritually stronger with each event in my life, living through such trials as epilepsy, brain surgery, recovery, and again death.

As I described how my studies and work as a counselor intern applied to my counseling abilities, I expressed my abilities to relate to clients and instill hope and faith by discovering their ability to persevere through their own storms in life. To overcome what they believed to be impossible, they developed a new perspective of themselves and focused on a life being filled with greater meaning by having a faith in God.

The staff reviewed my paper, and I received a passing grade. I was amazed at how fast five years had gone by and at the person I had become. There were moments I never believed I could have earned a master's degree, yet I did it.

The next step in practicing counseling was taking the state exam. The documentation and paperwork seemed to take forever. Then the day came to take the exam. This was much easier than taking the NCE, and it went very well. Within ten days, I received the letter with state certification; I was now a licensed graduate professional counselor (LGPC).

Section 7

New Beginnings

Chapter 18

The Engineer Retires

Retirement from a career does not mean the end to working; it is a new beginning to apply what you learn in life. Share your experience; you may bring hope to others.

My final couple of years with the Army Corps of Engineers involved sharing my knowledge by developing training programs. These programs were unique for I could give the various perspectives of the people needed to complete a project—the planner, designer, contracting officer, and construction representative. This was important in educating staff on the level of effort required and the decision-making process necessary to complete projects.

A young man who had worked with me for several years joked, saying, "It's okay for you to retire, for I'm not learning anything new from you anymore." He had become my right hand in helping with the training programs and was now doing the presentations. In fact, he was way ahead of me on formatting and resourcing presentations. His comment came at the perfect time because I had just turned in to the Human Resources Department the paperwork required for my retirement. I retired from the Army Corps of Engineers in the early fall.

Chapter 19

Epilepsy Advocacy

Advocacy is the ability to step forward and share personal experience and influence the perspective of a life situation for others.

It was time to relax and take some time off. My brain and body needed some rest after five years of working full time and studying for many hours each week. Retirement from the army corps and completing the curriculum at Loyola University left me with no work or school responsibilities. My pastoral counseling clinical work would start in January 2016. I continued to work as a mentor for the Chesapeake Chapter of the Epilepsy Foundation. Seems my free time would start to diminish as opportunities came along.

Through the Chesapeake Chapter came a recommendation to be trained in the UPLIFT program, developed by Emory University and funded through the Center for Disease Control and Prevention. (UPLIFT stands for Using Practice and Learning to Increase Favorable Thoughts.) This was a ten-week program starting in October focusing on helping groups of people diagnosed with epilepsy to manage stress. Upon completion, I was certified to facilitate groups of people, help them learn they are not alone in dealing with seizures, and develop skills to reduce stress in their lives.

Soon after this, I received a call from the Department of Defense, Peer Review Medical Research Program (PRMRP). Epilepsy research was now part of the medical research program, and they obtained my name through the Epilepsy Foundation. After the interview with the PRMRP staff, I was asked to become a consumer peer reviewer. They were excited about my joining the program and asked me to be a speaker at the kick-off dinner to talk about my own experience and the importance of the program. There would be many different professional review teams of various backgrounds. Several of the peers were asked to participate and, through personal example, express to the research reviewers the importance of the work they were about to perform.

I was relatively calm this time as I stood in front of sixty people consisting of doctors and researchers from all over the United States. Nine years earlier, I would have been visibly shaking with fear and would not have been capable of participating. My exposure to talking to and leading groups enabled my brain to rewire and build confidence.

The review board for the consumer advocacy was held in a hotel. I was very excited. When I arrived, my amygdala was fired up. As I walked across the parking lot from my car, my anxiety level increased. While this happened, another part of me was fascinated and interested in everything that was happening around me. Rooms were set up for meetings and advocates, and professionals came from all around the country. Some of the most interesting people were like me—the consumer advocates. I was handed the key to my room and my name tag for identification; everything was very well organized.

I needed to get to my room and drop off my bag of clothes needed for the three days of the review boards. As the doors to the elevator opened, I was overwhelmed with a strong smell of a cleaning fluid. It was identical to the smell of my room at Johns Hopkins Hospital, when I had my extended EEG. The hallway seemed bright, and the walls were white. The doors to the rooms looked just like the doors to the recovery rooms. It took a moment for me to realize I was looking down the hallway at the Johns Hopkins Hospital, yet this could not be possible. I felt my aura coming on and my heart beat getting faster.

In lieu of the panic attack and anxiety going to an extreme level, as it typically happened in the past, I was fascinated by what was happening inside of me. Through my studies to become a pastoral counselor, I had developed and utilized other channels of my brain to make up for the ones damaged or removed. I performed a self-analysis as a counselor and realized if fear and panic gained control,

I would lose consciousness. It was a session of countertransference within me. As I was evaluating and walking down the hallway, my heart beat returned to normal, and the aura stopped. The hallway was not at all like the hospital, for it was moderately lit with wood-finish paneling and a dark-colored carpet. I felt very tired, went into my room, and lay down to rest. I needed to be prepared for the evening events.

Everyone who was involved in a research review board was at the dinner and seated with the people they were to work with. Each team consisted of doctors and scientist from the most prestigious and known universities, hospitals, and research centers in the country. The room was filled with similar teams doing research on various diseases and recovery for the wounded soldiers. Epilepsy research was the latest to be funded, for seizures were becoming more common for the soldiers suffering from brain injury.

As we finished eating, the speakers were called up to the front of the room. When it was my turn, I walked up to the podium and looked over the people sitting at their tables. I was nervous and reminded myself of the importance of staying calm. I did fine reading the script I wrote until I read about my surgery. My mind became filled with fear of what had happened, and then I feared where I was. I had difficulty concentrating, and my brain shut down for a moment. To regain control, I took a deep breath, held it, and slowly let it out. I could feel myself begin to calm down and smiled, for such a simple action enabled me to regain control. My reading skills returned, and I completed the speech.

Everyone was moved by what they heard and gave me a standing ovation. When I got back to my table, the chief of the Epilepsy Review Board stood up and shook my hand and thanked me for speaking. He then went and got me dessert and something to drink. He noticed that I was having difficulty responding. I was not having a seizure—I was struggling with my emotions as I fought back tears. Once again, my emotions were based on my ability to do the impossible; it was another step forward in my recovery.

Through my studies, I learned it is not uncommon for someone having such experiences to become immobile or depressed. I had been down this path many times; however, this time I took on the role of a clinician and started to do a self-analysis. The counselor in Jon took over and was awed by learning how to control the uncontrollable within oneself. I smiled and thanked the Lord for the opportunity, not just to learn but also to understand how the mind works and our ability to reprogram. The engineer in me keeps working to determine the cause of a seizure. Most times there is no heart racing, only the sensation of the aura and anxiety triggered by seeing something similar to what was seen when I had a seizure. I am immediately reminded of what a seizure is like. When the aura is not strong, I wonder if it is even a form of a seizure or simply a memory of a dark time in my life.

My work as a licensed graduate professional counselor (LGPC) and coordinator started at the Westminster Rescue Mission a few weeks earlier than planned. Quite frankly, I was bored with my time off and was excited to start working as a clinician. The staff was a tremendous help in assisting me with my work and family life. My clinical work required being ready and willing to lead a group of men in a chapel as they found ways to overcome their addictions. Individual work was on a continuous basis. Helping men through the detoxification stage—from heroin and other drugs—required being available and willing to listen. Motivation came through other clients as they learned to be open with one another. Having a spiritual bond with God and understanding their role in life was most effective. Through this experience, I was learning the importance of counselor self-care to prevent burnout. Reminding myself that I was the messenger and the listener and not taking on the responsibilities of the client was extremely important.

Nine years after surgery, I was accepted into a training program at a hospital that prepares pastors in visiting patients. On the first day, we were given a tour of the hospital. I was nervous and wondering if I was ready. As we walked through the emergency care center, we saw many people seeking care. The beds and equipment reminded me of my own visits. Walking the OBGYN reminded me of the times my children were born, and I became anxious. At the end of the day, I asked the instructor if we could visit the emergency room again. More exposure was helping me recover.

As we approached one end of the emergency care center, we came across a family with an elderly parent who was dying. I watched the instructor in action and provided assistance. It seemed to come naturally, and I know that someday I will play that role too—just not yet.

Chapter 20

The End of Old and the Start of New Relationships

Knowing that there is a way it can be done is most effective in having the ability to overcome life challenges. This is when hope is implanted in you; little do you realize the day will come when someone else is struggling to climb the mountain of a life challenge and looks up and sees you. It is a way of instilling hope in others.

A relationship with someone dealing with seizures must be based on a love for the person, not on their possessions and not on just the good times. Rather, it is what you do when times get tough. Relationships can build, become closer and stronger during challenging times, and may be enhanced through the perspectives of those involved as individuals and family.

Unfortunately, the effect of serious health issues often leads to the end of a relationship. My relationship began to dissolve as my seizures slowly progressed and became intractable. Then my disability in remembering names and my brain shutting down when tired was frustrating. I felt alone in a battle that was driving us further apart. Home seemed to be the only place I did not want to be—too many memories of the hard times of my seizures, surgery, and recovery.

With the pressure of my counseling work and home life, it was time for my wife and me to separate. I moved out of the house, into an apartment, and into a new beginning. Eventually, I moved from the hectic fast-paced Baltimore/Washington area to the tranquil farm country of North Carolina, where some of my family lives. It was quite a change. However, I continue to work with the Epilepsy Foundation in Maryland and in North Carolina. I felt more at ease with the hassles of the metropolitan areas behind me. Little did I know there was a half marathon held here in support of people with epilepsy, and I would become a close friend and caregiver of someone I would fall in love with—someone recovering from a stroke and has seizures.

Chapter 21

Caregiving

The fundamentals of caregiving are listening, caring, asking, thanking, sharing, and learning.

The Role of the Mentor

A mentor is someone with real-life experiences who can help other people who are dealing with similar issues. As a mentor with the Epilepsy Foundation, I met many people diagnosed with epilepsy. Over time, I met their caregivers—typically the parents and spouses. There was a learning curve for me with every caregiver I met as each person was different in their knowledge of seizures, relationship with the individual they cared for, and control of their emotions and feelings. Many were overwhelmed by their fears and ignorance of seizures, especially those caring for someone recently diagnosed. The doctors provided excellent information concerning the medical treatment and resources; however, they were unable to give sufficient mental and emotional support.

Soon after volunteering to be a mentor, I received a call from a woman recently diagnosed with epilepsy. She was worried about how her two young children would react when she had a grand mal seizure. Her husband's shift work increased the time she would be alone with her children, and she wanted them to be prepared. Very young children suddenly had the responsibility of an adult.

During our training session, we talked about first aid and the responsibilities of the child caregiver. When I pretended to have a seizure, the younger child stayed with me as the older ran out of the room, screaming and close to panic state. She did grab the phone on her way out and called their father. When she returned to the room, she was sobbing, with tears streaming down her face as she feared her mother would die from a seizure.

Children can be strong when necessary. The expectation of what they should do is difficult to determine. They must know what is happening to their parent or sibling, who to contact for help, and the address of where they live. Access to a cell phone and knowing how to make the emergency call is most important. Cell phones today can give the position of the call to the EMS personnel, so be sure the GPS setting is activated.

Most importantly, caregivers, especially children, need attention when the seizure is over. They need to understand what happened, that they cannot control it, and that it is not their fault. It is amazing what young children conceive about a situation. Even my oldest son, at the age of two, recognized something was wrong with me and that I needed help sometimes. When he was a teenager, he had an uncanny ability to stay calm, contact emergency services, and know where to obtain the information the paramedics would need. His greatest fear was similar to the girl mentioned earlier—watching his father die from a seizure.

Education provided by people with experience is very effective in maintaining the appropriate perspective of epilepsy. Ignorance feeds fear in everyone and leads to isolation of the person with seizures. Isolation and fear leads to depression and losing hope. Mentors need to step forward and volunteer to help their peers and caregivers. Although I have earned a degree and license in counseling, being a mentor comes first.

Role of the Counselor

As a counselor working with the Maryland Chapter of the Epilepsy Foundation, I focused on helping those diagnosed with epilepsy. This was expanded to include the caregivers when I started working with Melanie whose daughter, Grace, for some unknown reason, had forty-four seizures in fifty-two days. While Grace was having seizures, Melanie would go for days without sleep and only slept a few hours when she did. Melanie's capability to function as a mother to Grace and her twin brother was impaired by her fears and love for her children.

For Grace, the doctors devised a treatment plan, involving some of the latest medications, to bring her seizures under control. However, the side effects of the medications changed her personality. Initially, her medication caused her to slow down and dampened her ability to perform in class. She was no longer the energetic little girl who was a whiz at math and reading. Her bright smile had faded, and she just functioned. She would eat little, could no longer learn anything, and suffered with depression. Her reading ability, which was outstanding for a child her age, diminished. And she could no longer remember her last name. Nothing could excite her, with the exception of the fear of having another seizure. She was no longer the little four-year-old who loved to read and play.

Over time, the doctors worked to find the most effective medication that would control Grace's seizures with minimal impact to her personality. Changing her medication and finding the appropriate dosage enabled her to regain some of her memory and participate with other children. For the next several months, it was difficult to determine if she was having absence seizures, a reaction to her medication, or just bored with class. Eventually, Grace came to one of our monthly group sessions. I struggled with my emotions as I talked with this beautiful little five-year-old girl. For her mother to watch her have so many seizures in such a short time must have been similar to having your soul torn away.

After eighteen months of treatment, Grace was taken off her medication because her EEG no longer indicated any seizure activity. She could laugh again! Her competency to learn increased significantly as her brain was no longer affected by medication.

Melanie appreciated the application of my insight to seizures with the sessions we had. Many of the sessions were held over the phone due to accessibility issues and time restraints. As I shared some of my experiences, she often said, "You need to share this." Melanie and Grace became my motivators to develop a five-week program for caregivers.

The Role of the Caregiver

The caregiver program includes first aid for the person with seizures and the caregiver, education about seizures and treatment, the perspective of the person with epilepsy, maintaining healthy relationships, and taking on challenges in a healthy manner. It is continually revised with each group as I learn more about the caregiver's perspective. Little did I know that one day I would become the caregiver of someone I loved and would witness her having seizures.

To minimize the stressors related to my work, and living near Washington, DC, I moved to a small town near the water in North Carolina. I did not know anyone, yet the people in the neighborhood were friendly, and I began to meet people throughout the community. I never expected to meet people with whom I had so much in common—Lori and James.

I like to run and was looking for a group to join. Upon researching for races in the area, I was shocked to see a half marathon and 5K race held every February in Washington, North Carolina. The person in charge of the program was James, who had seizures as a child that eventually became intractable. When he was seventeen, he had a lobectomy to regain control, and the surgery was very effective. Because he loves to run, he developed the *Race for Epilepsy Half Marathon/5K*. We had dinner together and surprised each other by how our experience with seizures and surgery were very similar.

Two weeks after moving to my new home, Lori moved into the house next door. She was also new to the area and knew only a few people through her work. The day she moved in, I was working in my yard and saw her approach me. As we chatted, I learned how much we had in common—sailing, fishing, and a second career in a ministry field. We both had suffered brain injuries; it had been six months since her stroke. She had recovered well; however, she had little sense of touch in her left arm and leg. I would not have noticed this if she had not pointed it out to me. She explained how she sometimes struggles with organizing thoughts and writing sentences—many similarities to my recovery from surgery. I was witnessing a miracle in motion as the doctors never thought Lori would survive her stroke, let alone be able to relocate and work at her career.

One evening, I heard the doorbell ring, and Lori was standing near the doorway. She apologized for interrupting me and said she needed help. When she came into the house, she asked me to look at her eyes. Her eyes were moving independently of each other even though she was trying to look straight at me. She said she saw one of her dogs run down the hallway in her house numerous times. In reality, the dog had gone down the hallway one time. Her brain just kept playing it over and over again. I was surprised she could see and comprehend enough to walk to my house. She was actually having a seizure, and I hurriedly drove her to the hospital. Later that evening, they transported her to another hospital with neurological care facilities and performed a twenty-four-hour EEG.

Over the next several months, we became closer friends. Not many people would get up and go fishing with me at 4:30 AM; however, Lori has many times. We have travelled to the Midwest, the Gulf Coast, and have sailed together. Although we have known each other for only a few months, it seems we have been best friends for many years.

Through her experience, Lori started to understand more about me. One evening, we were with some of my family, and she sensed something was amiss. No one else saw it. I had returned from a long trip that day and was very tired. For a moment, my expression flickered from smiling to a straight face as we walked down a hallway. I was having an aura that was triggered by exhaustion, dehydration, and being in a house that reminded me of the past. I was reacting to actually being back in that old home—in a dark place, with the smell of the old building. She saw it, yet no one else responded at the time. Even my sister did not realize what had just happened.

The challenge to both of us has been her seizures as they have become more intense and occur more often. There are times she has called or texted me with "I'm having a seizure!" Several times, I have watched as the seizures spread and become more acute, her body contracting and her face distorting. Throughout this, she can still hear what was happening around her. She said, "I feel safe when I hear your voice," because she knows I will take care of her.

Although I have seen many people have seizures, this was different. Now I was seeing a close friend have multiple partial and complex seizures and have an understanding of the emotional impact they have on a caregiver. In some ways, caring for her is easier because I can relate to what is happening. In other ways, it is difficult because I have lived through the trauma of having seizures myself. Watching her have an extended grand mal seizure has helped me realize what my caregivers lived through. Fortunately, I learned from Melanie and applied the techniques we shared in our caregiver program. I had to define my limits or reach the stage of burnout.[15] Burnout for me can lead to a relapse of my seizures. I had to accept I cannot stop her seizures. To be most effective, I have to take care of myself.

Lori is troubled by some people she works with because they expect her to perform 100 percent. They do not understand why she has difficulty, and they aggravate her situation by complaining she "looks" normal because her injury is invisible. Fortunately, the management is understanding and continues to work with her. To exacerbate the problem, there is no support system in the area for people recovering from stroke or dealing with seizures. For me, it is aggravating to watch someone come so far in recovery from a stroke and suffer such a setback due to seizures. She is enduring the situation as she learns how it takes time to develop an effective treatment.

---

[15]   For more information on Caregivers Care, see Appendix A.

Treatment includes finding a medication that is affordable since many of the new medications cost thousands of dollars a month.[16]

In spite of the seizures, we still do what we enjoy—being on the water and sailing. We love the ability to choose where we want to go, with the understanding we must be willing to adjust our course, as we have no control over the wind. The wind can suddenly change direction or drastically increase or decrease. Just like the impact of a seizure, we must be ready to adjust the sails or the course we are headed. We make a good team that can maintain control of the boat in any situation. When the storms come, we seek shelter and have backup systems to keep the boat at anchor and maintain a safe-haven.

Lori and I have talked about our life experiences and are aware that the most effective treatment in recovery from any situation is the ability to have a positive outlook and move forward. I refer to this as hope. Lori takes this a step further and refers to it as redemption.

---

[16] Often the outrageous cost of medical support and medications leads people to live with seizures that are preventable. Be sure to talk to your insurance company and your doctor about your ability to afford the cost of the medication being prescribed.

Epilogue

Seizures are a reminder about how fragile life is, and that life should be cherished.

Although I have written much about what it is like to live with epilepsy, it should be noted that it is a part of my life, not all of my life. I have been able to live a full and prosperous life because I search for meaning and refuse defeat. This is the engineer in me, who is always searching for solutions when facing challenges, and the counselor, who focuses on the positive. I like to smile and laugh, even when life is challenging and seems out of control.

I am no longer the nineteen-year-old who was warned by his father to keep quiet about my disability, because my disability became an ability I am blessed with. It enabled me to help people who were overwhelmed by what they were experiencing. Seizures are reminders about how fragile life is and that life should be cherished.

Writing this book started with often being told in my counseling courses, that I should share my story. It required reliving some of the darkest times in my life and facing those deep feelings of frustration, anger, defeat, and brokenness. Yet, with each event I wrote about, I felt stronger because those times helped me appreciate what I have been in training for; to inspire hope in others.

What carried me through my dark times has been a faith that God had a plan for me. It was nurtured through hope that there was meaning to what was happening. Seizures taught me that being a good leader requires relying on other people, being humble, and seeking the good in any situation.

My hope for those of you who are dealing with seizures is that you receive the help needed to control them. That there is a caregiver who is ready when needed and loves you for who you are. That you overcome the fear of a seizure and they become only a temporary set-back. May you still be able laugh and feel joy. The day may come when someone will look at you and be inspired by your experience and ability to live with such a disability. When that happens, you become a source of hope to other people.

Appendix A

When to Seek Emergency Assistance and to Call 911

There are five instances when you should call for emergency medical support (EMS):

1. If the seizure lasts more than five minutes, unless you know that the person's seizures typically last longer than five minutes. Remember, unless you are a primary caregiver who has been trained in the use of a special medication, or if you have been shown how to use a special VNS magnet, there is *nothing* you can do to stop a seizure—it will run its own course. You can protect the person from injury, observe the seizure, call for an ambulance if necessary, and reassure others that this is just a seizure and everything will be fine in a few moments.

2. The person has another seizure without regaining consciousness or is having difficulty breathing.

3. If they have other known medical conditions such as fever, diabetes, or is pregnant. Such conditions may be the cause or trigger of the seizure and require changes to the treatment plan.

4. The person suffers significant injury from the seizure, such as a broken bone or blow to the head, shoulders, or arms.

5. When you feel you need assistance. Watching someone have a grand mal seizure is not easy, and for some it is traumatic. This is especially true when the person having the seizure is bigger than the caregiver and moving them on their side or simply keeping them in a safe area requires assistance. Calling EMS does not mean the person must be transported to the hospital.

Basic Guide for the Caregiver

1. Don't panic! It shuts down your brain's ability to reason and respond appropriately.
2. Be aware that the individual may be able to see and hear what is happening.
3. Protect the head with a cushion, pillow, or soft object; your hands work well too.
4. Talk to the person throughout the stages of their seizure in a calm voice to reflect you care and are with them. Simple statements such as "Your safe. I am with you."
5. Allow the body to straighten. Arms and legs that are not able to straighten may lead to serious injury. Be careful when you do so. When releasing someone's leg from under a chair, they will kick very hard. Don't be in the way.
6. Seek emergency support when the following occurs:
   a. If the seizure last longer than five minutes (ictal state), seek emergency assistance.
   b. If the person has recurring seizures in a short period of time, seek medical assistance.
   c. If the seizure causes significant injury to the body or head.
   d. *You need the support to handle the situation.* When you have any doubts about the outcome, call 911. Remember, they will respond to provide emergency treatment and transport if they and you deem it necessary for additional medical support.
7. Set up a support system. Especially if you cannot lift the person. This can be a neighbor or close friend.
8. Keep a list of the medications, including dosage and time of day they are administered. Have a copy available to give to emergency personnel and those providing medical assistance or treatment.

9. Be prepared to give first aid to those who may witness the individual having a seizure.
10. You may also contact your local chapter of the Epilepsy Foundation to obtain training and information.

Be sure to take care of yourself!

Guidelines from the Epileptic's Perspective

The following is based on what I needed to pull me through. Negativity drives depression; find a way to be positive. Here are some key points to consider as the caregiver:

1. When I have a seizure, please be *aware* I may be able to see and hear what you do and say. Try to be *positive*.
2. Speak calmly. Tell me you *love* me.
3. Make this *our* battle, not my battle.
4. Be a part of my life, not a *critic* of my life.
5. Inspire me for what I have achieved in spite of my disability. *Laugh* with me.
6. Help me set high levels of recovery through setting *realistic* milestones. Then *cheer* me on.
7. All the other parts of the body when injured may take a few days to several months to heal. The brain requires years and a *desire* to do so.
8. Most importantly, *love me for who I am, not who you wished I could be.*

Appendix B

Epilepsy Support Agencies

Epilepsy Foundation
8301 Professional Place East, Suite 200
Landover, Maryland: 20785-2353
Phone: 301-459-3700
24/7 Epilepsy and Seizures Helpline: 1-800-332-1000
Spanish Speakers Only: 1-866-748-8008
Email: ContactUs@efa.org

Epilepsy Foundation, Maryland Chapter
Mary Wontrop, executive director: mwontrop@efa.org
8301 Professional Pl Ste 200
Landover, Maryland: 20785-2353
Phone: (301) 918-2100
Toll-free: (800) 332-1000

Epilepsy Foundation, North Carolina Chapter
Patricia A. Gibson, MSSW DHL ACSW
Director, Epilepsy Information Service
Associate professor, Department of Neurology
Wake Forest University School of Medicine
Piedmont One, Suite 5541 A
1920 West First Street
Winston Salem, North Carolina 27104
1-800-642-0500
Fax: 336-716-6018
pgibson@wakehealth.edu

Citizens United for Research in Epilepsy (CURE)
430 W. Erie, Suite 210
Chicago, IL, 60654
(312) 255-1801
1 (844) 231-2873 (toll-free)

People can learn more about Project UPLIFT from http://managingepilepsywell.org/programs/uplift.html.
If they want to know if there is someone trained to deliver Project UPLIFT in their state, there is a list of trained providers by state at the bottom of the page here: http://managingepilepsywell.org/programs/uplift_training.html

Appendix C

Types of Seizures

Some types of seizures include the following[17]:

Generalized seizures. Generalized seizures involve both sides of the brain. There is loss of consciousness and a postictal state after the seizure occurs. Types of generalized seizures include the following:

Absence seizures (also called petit mal seizures). These seizures are characterized by a brief altered state of consciousness and staring episodes. Typically, the person's posture is maintained during the seizure. The mouth or face may twitch, or the eyes may blink rapidly. The seizure usually lasts no longer than thirty seconds. When the seizure is over, the person may not recall what just occurred and may go on with his or her activities, acting as though nothing happened. These seizures may occur several times a day. This type of seizure is sometimes mistaken for a learning problem or behavioral problem. Absence seizures almost always start between ages four to twelve years.[18]

Atonic (also called drop attacks). With atonic seizures, there is a sudden loss of muscle tone, and the person may fall from a standing position or suddenly drop his or her head. During the seizure, the person is limp and unresponsive.

Generalized tonic-clonic seizures (GTC, or also called grand mal seizures). The classic form of this kind of seizure, which may

---

17   From the Johns Hopkins Medicine Health Library under nervous system disorders, epilepsy, and seizures.

18   Absence—the earlier childhood absences almost always remit by late childhood; the later childhood ones (e.g. age of onset six to eight) are called juvenile absences and usually continue and form tonic-clonic seizures in adulthood.

not occur in every case, is characterized by five distinct phases. The body, arms, and legs will flex (contract), extend (straighten out), and tremor (shake), followed by a clonic period (contraction and relaxation of the muscles) and the postictal period. Not all these phases may be seen in everyone with this type of seizure. During the postictal period, the person may be sleepy, have problems with vision or speech, and may have a bad headache, fatigue, or body aches.[19]

Myoclonic seizures. This type of seizure refers to quick movements or sudden jerking of a group of muscles. These seizures tend to occur in clusters, meaning they may occur several times a day or for several days in a row.

Infantile spasms. This rare type of seizure disorder occurs in infants before six months of age. There is a high occurrence rate of this seizure when the child is awakening or when he or she is trying to go to sleep. The infant usually has brief periods of movement of the neck, trunk, or legs that lasts for a few seconds. Infants may have hundreds of these seizures a day. This can be a serious problem and can have long-term complications that affect growth and development.

Febrile seizures. This type of seizure is associated with fever and is not epilepsy, although a fever may trigger a seizure in a child who has epilepsy. These seizures are more commonly seen in children between six months and five years of age, and there may be a family history of this type of seizure. Febrile seizures that last less than fifteen minutes are called simple and typically do not have long-term neurological effects. Seizures lasting more than fifteen minutes are called complex, and there may be long-term neurological changes in the child.

Focal or partial seizures. Focal seizures take place when abnormal electrical brain function occurs in one or more areas of one side of the brain. Focal seizures may also be called partial seizures. With

---

[19]   The bilateral tonic-clonic seizures are by far the most dangerous. They often cause brief postictal paralysis with impaired breathing. Those who have seizures out of sleep while facedown are at special risk for asphyxiation (SUDEP).

focal seizures, particularly with complex focal seizures, a person may experience an aura, or premonition, before the seizure occurs. The most common aura involves feelings, such as déjà vu, impending doom, fear, or euphoria. Visual changes, hearing abnormalities, or changes in the sense of smell can also be auras. Two types of focal seizures include the following:

Simple focal seizures. The person may have different symptoms depending on which area of the brain is involved. If the abnormal electrical brain function is in the occipital lobe (the back part of the brain that is involved with vision), sight may be altered, but muscles are more commonly affected. The seizure activity is limited to an isolated muscle group, such as the fingers, or to larger muscles in the arms and legs. Consciousness is not lost in this type of seizure. The person may also experience sweating, nausea, or may become pale.

Complex focal seizures. This type of seizure commonly occurs in the temporal lobe of the brain—the area of the brain that controls emotion and memory function. Consciousness is usually lost during these seizures. Losing consciousness may not mean that a person passes out—sometimes, a person stops being aware of what's going on around him or her. The person may look awake but may have a variety of unusual behaviors. These behaviors may range from gagging, lip-smacking, running, screaming, crying, or laughing. When the person regains consciousness, he or she may complain of being tired or sleepy after the seizure. This is called the postictal period.